T0246036

The
Story
of a
Heart

Two Families, One Heart,
and the Medical Miracle That
Saved a Child's Life

Dr. Rachel Clarke

Scribner
New York London Toronto Sydney New Delhi

Scribner
An Imprint of Simon & Schuster, LLC
1230 Avenue of the Americas
New York, NY 10020

First Scribner hardcover edition September 2024

SCRIBNER and design are trademarks of Simon & Schuster, LLC

Simon & Schuster: Celebrating 100 Years of Publishing in 2024

For information about special discounts for bulk purchases,
please contact Simon & Schuster Special Sales at 1-866-506-1949
or business@simonandschuster.com.

The Simon & Schuster Speakers Bureau can bring authors to
your live event. For more information or to book an event,
contact the Simon & Schuster Speakers Bureau at 1-866-248-3049
or visit our website at www.simonspeakers.com.

Interior design by Silverglass

Manufactured in the United States of America

1   3   5   7   9   10   8   6   4   2

Library of Congress Cataloging-in-Publication Data has been applied for.

ISBN 978-1-6680-4543-5
ISBN 978-1-6680-4545-9 (ebook)

TO KEIRA

A child whose kindness and compassion endure to this day

in the lives she is helping to save

Contents

Prologue ix

Keira 1

Max 19

Resuscitation 33

Crocodiles 49

Limbo 71

HeartWare 91

Matching 115

Waiting 133

Goodbye 145

Judgment 157

Retrieval 175

Transplant 189

Aftermath 205

Epilogue 215

Acknowledgments 219

Notes 221

Prologue

This is the tale of a boy, a girl, and the heart they share. It is a story that no one was meant to tell. In the impassioned world of transplant surgery, the families of organ donors almost never encounter the people into whom those organs are transplanted. For obvious reasons, transplant services go to great lengths to ensure that donor and recipient families are kept at a distance. The entire process of organ donation is fraught enough without creating additional emotional entanglements that could heap distress upon vulnerable individuals.

Exceptionally rarely, however, donor and recipient families do discover each other's identity. Invariably the catalyst is media attention. I first encountered the story of nine-year-old Max Johnson in the *Mirror*, in June 2017. In England at that time, people who wished to donate their organs after death had to proactively opt *in* to making their wishes known by signing up to the national organ donor register. Many medical and patient advocacy groups argued that more lives could be saved if the law was changed so that—as in a growing number of other countries—adults would be presumed to have consented to organ donation unless they opted *out*. The hope was that this would address the scarcity of organs, enabling many more lives to be saved. The *Mirror*, a newspaper with a history of advocating on a wide range of social issues, chose to run a campaign on this one. Under the headline "Change the Law for Max," the paper ran a front-page splash making a powerful appeal to the then UK prime minister Theresa May to introduce new legislation addressing the scarcity of organs available for transplant.[1] The editor hoped that public pressure would galvanize the government into making the drafting of the necessary legislation a priority.

Max had been a soccer-playing, tree-climbing, play-fighting force of nature until a mysterious illness caused his heart to fail, leaving it so dangerously weak and unstable he was forced to spend nine months confined to a hospital bed. Ordinarily, nothing in the human body is quite as single-minded as the heart. Its four chambers, fibrous flesh, electrical waves, and swing-door valves are designed with one aim and one alone: to beat. Through beating—or, more accurately, through contracting then relaxing—the muscle of the heart jolts blood into every last crevice of the human body, delivering oxygen, nutrients, and hormones to tissues, while whisking away the cellular by-products of life. Around 100,000 times a day—3 billion times over an average lifetime—all four chambers squeeze as one, forcing blood to surge through our arteries. The adult heart pumps 260 liters of blood every hour, enough to fill a small swimming pool each day. One contraction is so powerful it can send blood spurting ten feet straight up into the air if the aorta, the body's principal artery, is severed. The heart, in short, is a toiling, tireless, muscular miracle. Barely the size of a pair of clasped hands, its capacity for circulating blood is extraordinary.

Max's heart muscle had been fatally harmed, probably by a mild viral infection he had scarcely noticed. While Max was in the hospital, his parents acquired the new and terrible knowledge that up to one in five children in Britain and America might die while waiting on the transplant list. They were equally aware that the only thing that could give Max what he needed to live was the death, appallingly, of someone else's child. Max became the poster boy for the

Mirror's campaign. Young, sweet, and immensely charismatic, he captivated the hearts of readers. After months of waiting for a replacement heart—and just when it started to seem that hope was lost—another child, Keira, had the terrible misfortune to suffer a catastrophic brain injury as a result of a road traffic collision. Keira's family, upon being told she was brain dead, immediately decided to gift her organs. They knew with absolute certainty that this was what their daughter would have wanted.

In September 2017, a photo of Max in his hospital bed dominated the front page of the *Mirror* once more.[2] The former wraith whose haunted stare had so moved readers was now pink-cheeked and beaming. His chest was bandaged, hiding a livid median sternotomy scar that extended all the way from the top of his sternum to the bottom of his ribs. Behind that scar, Keira's heart sat and squeezed, flooding his body with blood and life. In addition to Max, Keira's organs had saved the lives of another child and two adults. Overwhelmed with gratitude, Max's parents, Emma and Paul Johnson, shared the following letter with the UK's transplant service, NHS Blood and Transplant, who gave it in turn to the anonymous child's family:

> *To the donor family,*
>
> *We are writing to you as you hold a very special place in our hearts. Our son, Max, is 9 and he had a heart transplant. He was very poorly and a heart transplant was his only chance of coming home and starting a new life.*
>
> *We are so sorry that you lost your loved one, but we would like to thank you for the incredibly kind, courageous decision that you made to allow organs to be donated. We do not know the circumstances, but we can only imagine what a dreadful, harrowing time you have been through and are doubtless still going through, with the loss.*

Even in your grief, you have made a selfless decision to help others and we are indescribably grateful to you.

We hope that it brings you some comfort to know that Max's post-transplant recovery has been smooth and without complication. His new heart has been described as a happy heart and a brilliant heart. Max is very thankful and he is looking after his new heart. He says "Good Morning" to his new heart every day and sends it lots of love, while it adjusts to the new environment.

He is eating healthily and exercising when he feels able, so that his heart will stay fit and strong. Max is getting used to all the medication, but he is full of energy and enthusiasm, as a result of the new lease of life that has been gifted by your family. He is relishing every moment back at home, without sickness, tubes, wires, machines, procedures etc. It was a very upsetting time, waiting so long for the call, but when we did get the call, we prayed for you and your family.

We continue to pray for you and think about you. We wanted you to know that your sacrifice was not in vain and you have given an incredible legacy of love and good will to others. We thank you so much for making a decision that has saved our son and given him the prospect of a future ahead of him. As he grows older, we will encourage him to cherish his heart in memory of you.

With our eternal gratitude,
Emma and Paul

When Keira's parents received this letter, they realized that the Max to whom it referred was very likely to be the same Max whose plight they had read about in the *Mirror*. It took no time at all for Keira's mother, Loanna, to locate Emma Johnson on Facebook. After much deliberation, Loanna decided to write a letter of her own, introducing herself via a private message to the mother of the boy whose life her daughter had almost certainly saved. What happened next would change the history of transplant surgery in the UK.

———

Organ transplantation is both a marvel of modern medicine and one of the purest expressions of human altruism. In 2022 alone, the lives of 42,887 people in the US were saved by the generosity of 21,369 people donating their organs after death.[3] Collectively, over a million lifesaving transplants have been successfully performed in the US since records began. In the UK, the numbers are smaller but still remarkable. In 2022, organs donated by 1,429 people after their death saved the lives of 3,575 people.[4] Right now, there are currently over 60,000 people alive in Britain—planning their child's birthday party, setting off on a bike ride, enjoying an ice cream, savoring the summer sun—thanks to the gift of another person's heart, liver, kidney, or lungs.[5] Without this radical generosity, the vast majority of those individuals would be dead. None of them would be alive without the doggedness, toil, and creative genius of a remarkable cast of doctors and scientists whose obsession and brilliance in the twentieth century led to the series of medical breakthroughs that enabled the death-defying act of removing an organ from one human body and successfully reimplanting it in another.

Transplant surgery today is conducted with such skill and rigor that almost no part of the anatomy is too challenging to replace. Bones, tendons, heart valves, veins, voice boxes, uteruses, penises, nerves, and entire limbs have all successfully been transplanted. In 2008, a thirty-eight-year-old woman in the UK gave birth to the world's first baby from a transplanted ovary.[6] Two years later, the first total face transplant—comprising skin, muscles, eyelids, nose, lips, upper and lower jaw, teeth, palate, and cheekbones—was performed on a man in Spain who had been severely disfigured in a shooting accident.[7] Since then, bilateral arm and leg transplants have occurred, unmanned drones have delivered donor kidneys to patients in remote hospitals, and lifelong illnesses such as sickle cell disease and type 1 diabetes have been cured by transplants of bone marrow[8] and insulin-producing pancreatic islet cells,[9] respectively.

The hidden logistics required to ensure no viable organ goes to waste are immense. Most moderate- and high-income countries have a national organ register and transplantation service that co-ordinates the retrieval, distribution, and transplantation of organs according to fairness and need.

The UK's National Organ Retrieval Service comprises sixteen teams of exceptionally skilled surgeons, anesthesiologists, and the-ater operatives. At any given moment, day or night, 365 days a year, up to eleven of these teams can plunge into action, retrieving pre-cious organs from hospitals anywhere in the country. The alloca-tion of organs is determined by the NHS Organ Donor Register, established after a lengthy campaign by two bereaved parents, John and Rosemary Cox, who fought for their twenty-four-year-old son, Peter, to become a donor after he died of a brain tumor in 1989.[10] In the midst of their grief, the Coxes were dismayed to discover that no national register existed of people who wanted to donate their organs after their death. They wrote hundreds of letters, gave multiple newspaper and television interviews, and tirelessly lobbied the government until, in 1994, the register was finally set up. Today, more than 30 million people are registered, representing 42 percent of the UK population.[11]

Underpinning both the positioning of patients on the waiting lists for organs and the logistics of organ procurement is rigorous science. Every human organ is delicately embedded in a cat's cradle of veins, arteries, nerves, and tissues that sustain and control its function. Less than a century ago, the idea of surgically excising a human organ, transporting it on ice, and successfully implanting it into another living person's body was the stuff of science fiction. Children in end-stage organ failure today stand a chance at life thanks to decades of laborious effort and flashes of inspiration from immunologists, vascular surgeons, physiologists, pharmacologists, anesthesiologists, engineers, and many other doctors and scientists. An entirely new medical specialty—intensive care—had to be invented before transplantation could occur successfully, not to mention the small matter of redefining the very concept of death itself.

Sustaining the science of transplantation is something equally wondrous: the human instincts that underpin every donation. There is no purer act of giving. The impulse to donate your organs after death, or those of your child, arises from the desire—as profound as it is simple—to help a fellow human being, irrespective of who they are or where they come from. Grieving relatives will often derive immense comfort from the knowledge that the person they once loved so dearly has, through their death, enabled others to live, but this does not diminish a donor or a donor family's fundamental altruism.

As with all medical advances, however, the new technologies of transplantation expose uncomfortable truths and ethical dilemmas. Organs are inherently scarce. Therefore, as moral philosopher Janet Radcliffe Richards says in her elegant book on the subject, *The Ethics of Transplants*: "to put the matter objectively and starkly, there is a perpetual competition between the people who need organs and the rest of us who have them. We are all now potential sources of spare parts for people whose own organs have failed, and whose hope lies in getting one of ours."[12]

At its ugliest, this conflict is played out in horror stories from around the world about black-market organ trafficking. In Afghanistan, for example, after the Taliban returned to power in 2021, crushing poverty and famine forced displaced, starving people to sell both their children and their body parts. At the time, the going rate for a kidney was around 150,000 afghani or just over £1,000 (a daughter could be sold for less than half this price).[13] In China, despite official denials, evidence exists of systematic, state-sanctioned, involuntary harvesting of kidneys and portions of livers from prisoners while they are still living, plus the macabre phenomenon of "execution by organ procurement" in the case of those incarcerated on death row, whose organs are harvested prior to, not after, their slaughter.[14] It is tempting to recoil from the amorality of this trade in stolen body parts. Kazuo Ishiguro, in his devastating novel *Never Let Me Go*, chooses instead to confront and interrogate the psychology of a world in which children are cloned and bred for the sole purpose of harvesting their organs once they reach adulthood.[15] His fictional dystopia forces us to consider how fiercely we yearn to extend our own lease on life, and—perhaps even more uncompromisingly—the life span of those we love.

Several thousand people die in the UK and the US every year while hoping and waiting for a donor organ, the clock inexorably ticking down. The donors from whom organs are euphemistically "sourced" or "made available" are, of course, human beings themselves, with all the ethical consequences that entails. Radcliffe Richards makes the assumption that:

> The people on the waiting list for transplants from deceased donors are, in effect, hoping that one of the rest of us will die so that they can have our organs. And, furthermore, their hopes are not for the incidental scraps left behind by those of us who have reached the inevitable end of a long life, because if we die from the wearing out of our own body parts they will not be of much use to anyone else. What the patients hoping for transplants

need, ideally, is the sudden death of a young and healthy person, whose organs are still in good condition.[16]

Yet for those waiting for organs and their families there is a subtle but incredibly important distinction. Far from "wishing" that someone else's child will die, their only hope is that—should another family find themselves in the unthinkable situation of losing a child—they might find it within themselves to say yes to organ donation going ahead.

Moreover, these moral complexities ensure that organ donation is rightly one of the most tightly regulated areas of modern medicine. It is crucial that the instinctive altruism underpinning a person's decision to donate their own organs after their death, or those of a deceased family member, is not in any way tainted by the suggestion that doctors are seeking to retrieve organs through opportunistic or self-serving means. The medical teams who treat patients and diagnose death are deliberately kept entirely separate from the teams responsible for organ donation. Nobody in the UK or US is paid for their organs. Nor do clinicians or managers profit from arranging an organ retrieval. These are not transactions of power or of wealth. They are exchanges whose driving force is compassion. They reflect the startling capacity of death's proximity to strip away life's trivial details. If we allow ourselves to consider, for a moment, our final days, could anything befit them more than helping to save—through death—the life of another human being? How could we resist such radical kindness?

———

I am not a surgeon but a physician who specializes in palliative care, the branch of medicine in which matters of life and death are more

intricately entwined than any other. I became captivated by the wonder of transplant surgery during my pediatrics rotation at medical
school. I had just returned to my studies after a year's maternity
leave. My son was at the age where everything—airplanes, trucks,
cobwebs, bananas—was intoxicating. He stampeded more than tod-
dled, roared when excited, and routinely laughed with such gusto he
would tip himself onto the floor. The fear and anguish endured by
the parents I met on the children's ward was painful to witness.

One day, I accompanied one of the hospital's most experienced
pediatric cardiologists on his morning ward round. Tall and griz-
zled, an elder statesman of the children's hospital whom I will call
Dr. Brewer had three decades of expertise in the medicine of keeping young hearts beating. We entered the room of a young boy,
perhaps ten or eleven years old. "Hello, Ben. Hello, Gary," said
Dr. Brewer to the child and his distraught-looking father, whose
names, again, I have changed. As Dr. Brewer crouched down so as
not to tower over Ben, the crack of his knees filled the room. Ben's
bedsheets were strewn with untouched electronic detritus—iPad,
headphones, mobile. A tub of sweets sat unopened on the bedside
table. His body was limp, eyes barely focused. His pale face was
sheened in sweat, and beneath the condensation fogging the oxygen mask, his lips were unmistakably blue. Ben, like Max Johnson,
was in acute heart failure. A viral infection had caused the muscle
of his heart to weaken so catastrophically it could no longer pump
effectively. Blood no longer raced through his arteries, but clogged
and distended the veins of his body and lungs, which were, by now,
so waterlogged that Ben could barely breathe.

"How are you feeling today?" Dr. Brewer asked gently.

"Okay," whispered Ben—a transparent lie.

"What now?" asked Gary as his son's eyelids fluttered and closed.
The hospital's cardiologists and cardiothoracic surgeons were locked

in a dispute about how best to manage Ben's condition. Although he had been placed on the waiting list for an urgent heart transplant, he had deteriorated to such an extent that he needed immediate mechanical assistance—an artificial metallic pump to supplement the dwindling efforts of his heart to beat. The experts were wrangling over which device was best.

"I will speak to the surgeons and come back to see you this afternoon," said Dr. Brewer. "We need to sort this out today."

A short while later, the ward round complete, I was heading back to the lecture hall when two doctors sped past at a sprint. Their pagers crackled and a telephonist barked: "Pediatric crash call. Pediatric crash call. Proceed to Robin Ward, Room Three." I stopped in my tracks. It was Ben's room.

Inside the darkness of the lecture hall, news spread and somebody whispered, "God, did you hear about that boy with dilated cardiomyopathy on Robin?" Ben had suffered a cardiac arrest minutes after we left his bedside. The crash team had been unable to restart his heart and he died as his father looked on. When I left the hospital at the end of the day, I happened to pass Dr. Brewer. He looked older, diminished, and freighted with sorrow. We hovered awkwardly in the corridor. "I'm so sorry," I mumbled. He nodded slowly before turning away, his eyes filling with tears.

Those scenes are as vivid to me today as when I first witnessed them. A transplant snatches life from death. Depending on your point of view, the transplantation of a human heart is a miracle, a violation, a leap of faith, an act of sacrilege. It's a dream come true, a death postponed, a biomedical triumph, a day job. Perhaps it is all these things simultaneously. One thing is abundantly clear, though. Transplant surgery, more than any other branch of medicine, poses ethical questions of immense importance. How, for example, does any parent contemplate their child's heart pumping while their brain is dying? How do they face the prospect of another child seeing through their own child's eyes, or of breathing through their lungs? Does the act of removing one person's organs and implanting them into another's body not so much push at as transgress the boundaries of being human? What does it cost a healthcare professional to sit beside a grieving parent and first broach the topic of donating their child's organs? And how does a parent reconcile the flood of relief that a transplant may save their child with the guilt of knowing that this comes at the cost of another child's life? Questions like these propel the narrative of this book. Those of us who have never had to ask them are lucky indeed.

———

As soon as I learned about Max and Keira's story, I was captivated by the way in which their lives became entwined around a single, shared heart. From the moment Keira was fatally injured, her heart began a journey so momentous it was scarcely believable. First, there were the emergency chest compressions at the scene of the crash—a junior doctor's palms bearing down with all their might, striving to keep oxygen flowing through her body. Next, the strange metaphysical limbo between life and death as Keira lay in intensive care, warm, flushed, apparently sleeping, yet somehow—unfathomably—brain dead. Then the moment when her heart was stilled by an anesthesiologist's drugs so that the surgeons, silently at work within the cave of her chest, no longer faced a moving target. From there, the light aircraft dash halfway across the country to deliver the organ, chilled on ice, into gloved and poised surgical hands. Finally, the intricate knitting of the heart's great vessels into another child's torso—and the agonizing wait, every second an ordeal, to see if its chambers would resume their vital work.

I knew there was only one way I wanted to tell this extraordinary story: by placing the heart itself center stage. When Keira's heart defied nature to traverse time and space from one body to another, it affected the lives of all those involved in its journey—parents, siblings, surgeons, nurses, paramedics, bystanders, organ donation teams, pilots, psychologists, cardiologists. I set out to re-create this journey as faithfully as possible by writing, in essence, the biography of Keira's heart. Over the last four years I have interviewed each of the key individuals whose interventions enabled Keira's heart to resume its beat inside Max's body. Nothing is fictionalized or based on conjecture. Anything appearing in direct quotes was recorded by me in a formal interview, either in person or via video or a phone call. I have edited quotations as little as possible, and only for grammar or clarity. The dialogue in the book is based on the recollections of the people interviewed. Woven alongside the journey of Keira's heart is the broader historical story of how a dazzling array of biomedical achievements throughout the twentieth century enabled modern transplant surgery.

I have tried, in short, to write as complete an account as possible of the wonder and anguish, the science and soul, of a single heart in transit. This is Keira's heart. And here is its story.

Keira

Keira. A name that takes flight, like the cry of a bird. Just right for the child who here and now is slicing through sky, as near as flying herself, laughing out loud with the joy of it. Her horse Charlie's hooves are thumping on the turf. The fields pour past, the farm is a blur, the trees are molten.

At nine years old, your whole world is the present. Keira beams with delight, giddy, exultant, as somewhere beneath the grip of her thighs an equine heart opens, closes, opens, a liter of blood punched out with each contraction. Keira giggles and grins. She can't contain her excitement. When riding her horse, she's an arrow, a hawk. A child alight with the act of living.

When Keira returns to the yard from her ride, her mother, Loanna, finds herself grinning, too. How could you not be enchanted by this child's smile? With her face still pink and her own heart still racing, Keira wraps her arms around Charlie's neck. Her hair, light-colored, almost golden, falls in gleaming waves down her back. She leans in closer, pressing her cheek to the dampness of his coat, and whispers, praises. *Good boy, Charlie. Good boy.*

For the next hour at least, Loanna knows, her daughter will vanish inside the stables. It's an open secret within the family that Keira loves looking after Charlie even more than she loves riding him. Caring, loving, soft, gentle. Anyone who knows her describes the child in these terms. Notably, Keira is so besotted by animals she cannot walk past an overturned snail without having to stop and right it. A glass jar sits on her bedside table, home to displaced beetles, spiders, and other rescued invertebrates. She dreams of one day working with animals. Her favorite color is bright clown fish orange.

Don't be too long, Loanna calls after her daughter as Keira leads Charlie away from the paddock. It's late July—summer vacation time—and tonight the family has plans. Husband and wife, Joe and Loanna Ball, are taking Keira and her younger brother, Bradley, aged seven, to enjoy fish and chips on Barnstaple beach. Their two older children—Katelyn, age eleven, and Keely, age twelve—are having a sleepover with their auntie. It's getting late. Already the hillside is gilded with early-evening sunshine.

Much of Britain is rightly called beautiful, but swaths of Devon are irresistible. Every year the sea cliffs, sandy beaches, wild coves, and rolling pastures entice vacationing families and retirees in the thousands. Barnstaple, the north Devon coastal town where Keira lives with her family, stands on rich, dark soil on which dairy herds have flourished for centuries. The children's summer vacations are an open-air idyll on their grandparents' farm. They tend the horses, collect eggs from the chicken coop, run riot.

The cool recess of the stable is a welcome respite from the heat of midsummer. In the darkness Keira has no concept of time as she croons and chatters to Charlie. She fills a bucket with water and watches with undisguised pleasure as he guzzles it dry. Next, she unbuttons his saddle and tack, the leather stiff and unyielding to diminutive fingers. With a currycomb she loosens the dirt on his coat, working methodically, lovingly, from ear to tail. Now the dandy brush, to sweep away any debris. The horse nickers contentedly as the bristles dig deep, nodding and shuffling his pleasure. To Keira, these scents—sawdust, sweat, and the sweetness of hay—are the smell of home. She whistles and hums, so absorbed in her task she is unaware of the stable dust glinting around them.

The next morning—Sunday, July 30, 2017, at eleven o'clock precisely—everything is going to change. Later, and for the rest of her life, Loanna will keep returning to this moment. What will sit at the core of her, needling, taunting, is how outlandish the odds were. If events had aligned only fractionally differently, perhaps it all could have been undone. Suppose, for example, if Keira and Bradley, when offered the treat of a day out with Mum, had chosen the beach instead of learning how to leap through urban environments at junior parkour? Or if Loanna had decided not to take a detour, en route to the concrete park, to pick up a few supplies from a farm shop? Or—the most minuscule and therefore brutal tweak of all—if she had simply left the house one, two, three seconds later. Anything to take her car off that precise road, at that precise time. You could lose your mind just thinking about it.

The truth, though, as the forensic collision investigators will know the moment they are told the name of the road in question, is that for Keira the odds were rigged from the outset. The location of the crash—a section of the A361, also known as the North Devon Link Road—is infamous, both locally and nationally. In 2019, according to the UK Road Safety Foundation, this twenty-six-mile stretch of tarmac had the dubious accolade of being the tenth most dangerous rural road in Britain.[1] Fatal collisions occur here with astonishing frequency. Local media regularly list the names of the dozens of people who have been killed on the A361 since 2000, while road safety campaigners single it out as one of the small number of "persistently high-risk" roads that the government must urgently focus on improving to cut fatality rates.[2] Its most obvious flaw is the short passing lanes that merge with little notice, leading frustrated drivers into risky attempts at getting past slower vehicles. Each new fatality generates a clamor in Devon for upgrades and proper divided highways, but the necessary funding is never forthcoming.

The result is that even as it carves its way through some of the most beautiful countryside in the whole of England, the A361 is a twenty-six-mile minefield. Indeed, the very next day after the crash involving Loanna's car, two more vehicles will collide on the same stretch of road.[3] Almost inconceivably, another mother, Jane Baker-Lockett, and two more children, twelve-year-old twins James and Amy, will be killed when their car hits a semitruck. Three years after those children perish, works to improve the North Devon Link Road will finally be approved by the Department for Transport—though they have still not been completed at the time of writing.

———

Upon waking on July 30, 2017, Dr. Nick Hillier has every right to feel a little pleased with himself. In three days' time—the first Wednesday in August—he is at last going to become a fully registered medical practitioner, after twelve grueling months as a "pre-registration," or probationary, doctor. Every year on so-called Black Wednesday, Britain's gargantuan National Health Service creaks, groans, and steels itself for chaos, as some fifty thousand doctors-in-training move en masse from their old posts into new, unfamiliar medical rotations.[4] For patients, it is a time of not inconsiderable jeopardy. The most fearful and ill-equipped of these migrating doctors are the least qualified, the seven thousand or so final-year medical students who are taking their first qualified steps onto hospital wards. Never before have they treated patients unsupervised. Some of the profession's old-timers warn their families to steer clear of hospitals in early August if they can possibly help it.

For Nick, all this feels like ancient history. He has survived—better yet, excelled in—his first year as a doctor. With stellar feedback from his mentors and seniors, Nick has the world of medicine at his fingertips. Yet he isn't smug. Perhaps his decision to study medicine as a mature student has left him better acquainted than most of his peers with how remorselessly fate can punish over-confidence. It does not take very much medical practice to realize that no matter how nonchalantly we plot and plan, how cocooned in comfort or wealth we feel, each of us is a candidate for sudden extinction. Slips, trips, accidents, aneurysms, ice, knives, clogged arteries, roof tiles. Fate fells lives in their prime as cleanly as timber, and nothing ever truly protects us.

Tall and lean with thick-lashed eyes and a gentle demeanor, Nick has learned enough during his first year of medicine to recognize he is no longer the same as other people. "My first job was on a surgical admissions ward where loads of the patients got sick and died," he says. "When you're new and you get to know patients who don't make it, that's the beginning of your brutalization as a doctor. Then you get more brutalized by the mad stuff that goes on, the crazy stuff. When I was on-call at night there was never anyone more senior to help us. No registrars, no consultants. We didn't know what we were doing; we just had to learn as we went. It was wild. People died. I'd start CPR [cardio-pulmonary resuscitation] and it wouldn't be that different to the simulations you do at med school—except that in real life when you do CPR on someone you might break all their ribs, and then they die. That doesn't happen with a mannequin."

New doctors often talk like this, with the slightly shell-shocked air of a soldier just back from their first tour of duty. As Nick puts it, part of the point of your first year as a doctor is to be exposed to enough death, enough mess, enough trauma that they no longer affect your ability to perform under pressure. Instinct and emotion must be bludgeoned away. Otherwise, how will you act decisively, instead of flailing blindly, when confronted with a patient whose life hangs in the balance? It can be a dehumanizing apprenticeship, which not every new doctor survives.

That morning, though, Nick isn't giving medicine a second's thought. He and his partner, Sam, a biomedical scientist and healthcare assistant, have spent the week on vacation. Soporific, sun-drenched days of sand and surf have wiped hospital wards clean from Nick's mind. It's still early. He glances up sleepily at the bedroom window. Apart from the niggling prospect of the two-hundred-mile motorbike ride from Barnstaple back home, he feels as empty and serene as the cloudless sky. Already the day is beautiful.

———

Several miles from Nick and Sam's bedroom, a local farmer, William Paddon, has been fretting for hours. One of his prize cows is unwell and William waits, urging the creature to rally. Eventually, he attaches an eight-foot trailer to his Ford Ranger 4×4 pickup and prepares to take the animal to the vet for emergency treatment. At over sixteen feet long and two tons in weight, the Ford Ranger is marketed with the bullish slogan "Let Nothing Stand in Your Way."

———

Loanna Ball's kitchen is cheerful bedlam.

Joe! The toast!

Chocolate pillows! We want chocolate pillows!

Love you, Keira! Don't fall off the parkour!

Smoke billows from the toaster, Joe hunts for his mobile, and Keira and Bradley squeal into an iPad at their two older sisters while stuffing their mouths with their favorite breakfast cereal, the squares of cocoa and wheat they nicknamed chocolate pillows.

Come straight to the farm as soon as you've finished, Katelyn tells Keira. From the moment her younger sister was born, the two girls have been inseparable, blessed with the same vivacity and charm; a connection so fierce it seems impenetrable, otherworldly, to outsiders.

I will! Keira yells back into the screen. *And then we'll take the horses out!*

Their father, Joe, another lover of motorbikes, is dressed top to toe in his leathers. He, too, has several hundred miles of biking ahead of him. Today is the commemoration bike ride from Barnstaple to Bristol that Joe and a group of fellow bikers undertake every year to celebrate the life of a friend who died some years ago in a motorbike collision. A big, burly security guard, Joe's bulk belies the softness he shares with his youngest daughter. *Be good for Mum*, he instructs the children, then stoops to ruffle Bradley's and Keira's hair, kissing them goodbye with the ease of someone who dispenses affection un-stintingly, and who believes he has all the time in the world.

The die is cast. Everyone emerges into dazzling sunshine. Four keys turn in their locks, four engines turn over. Joe is gone in a blast of dust and leather while a pickup truck, a motorbike, and a white Vauxhall Vectra set out on their fatal convergence. Seagulls drift, traffic builds, toddlers whine, fingertips drum on sticky steering wheels. Time still flows. The world, if briefly now, remains ordered.

Are we there yet?

She pinched me.

I forgot my out-of-office.

Stop it. I won't tell you again.

Where's the sea?

I asked Geoff to water the garden.

Can we have an ice cream?

Did you remember to turn off the water?

Ordinary life, lazily unspooling, in the sweaty fug of a thousand cars snaking their way across North Devon. Somewhere in the speeding traffic, Keira and Bradley bicker over a packet of crisps. Nick computes which service station to stop at for petrol later. The cow lurches miserably in the back of its trailer. Locked in their trajectories, each vehicle approaches the point on the road—not yet notorious, not yet memorialized with tattered teddy bears and bunches of wilted flowers—where time will buckle and cave.

It is Sam, Nick's partner, who sees the smoke first. Without warning, both lanes of traffic are suddenly stationary. Head down, focused on the road ahead, Nick cautiously weaves through the gaps in the cars, while Sam looks ahead toward an ominous column of gray in the distance. "There were a lot of vehicles backed up all the way down the road," they say. "Being on the motorbike, we started filtering through, obviously wondering why this random road was suddenly at a standstill. I just remember thinking what you usually do when you see, like, an accident on the road, you know, don't rubberneck, don't look, just go on, don't contribute to the problem."

Nick and Sam near the collision. "It didn't look good. We saw some people milling about, and there'd clearly been a horrendous head-on crash between two vehicles," says Nick. "There was a trailer on a van with this unhappy-looking cow staring out of it, and a wreck of a car with smoke coming out.

They pull over. It dawns on them both that no emergency services are present. Clearly the collision has only just happened. Apart from several untrained members of the public clustered uncertainly around Loanna's car, there is nobody to help the casualties. Nick and Sam approach. Both, in theory, have vital skills to offer, but although Sam has been in their job as a healthcare assistant for over six months, they have only ever been taught basic life-support skills on a plastic mannequin. "They still hadn't got around to giving me the proper training. I didn't have any real training for this situation at all," they say. Nick, meanwhile, is undeniably proficient in advanced life-support skills, but the emergencies he is used to at work are controlled and clinical—patients in hospital beds with their vital signs monitored and crash teams ready to swoop in and save them. This is entirely different. There is heat, smoke, rising panic, floundering. Nobody with a clue what to do. As soon as the other bystanders learn Nick is a doctor they turn to him, distraught and frantic.

What do we do?

Tell us what to do.

Instinctively the pair begin to triage the casualties. Sam heads to the front of the car where Loanna and Bradley are at least able to speak. "Loanna was sort of crushed by the metal. She had just become one with the car. She was suspended, completely crushed. And she was groaning. I remembered that was good. I was like, 'Cool, she's making a noise,'" says Sam. Bradley, meanwhile, is white with blue lips. "He was obviously hurt, you could tell. I was like, 'How are you feeling? Are you cold?' And he said, 'Yeah, I feel cold.' 'Do you have any pain?' I asked. And he said, 'Yes, my chest,' and he was obviously in shock, so I just gave him my hoodie and started talking complete crap for him, things like 'Oh, I've got a friend called Bradley.' I was trying to keep him calm and distract him. I just didn't want him to look at his mum."

Bradley, doctors will later discover, is losing blood from a ruptured spleen. His seat belt is acting as a temporary tourniquet, arresting the hemorrhage that might otherwise kill him. As Sam wraps the little boy in their hoodie, willing him to stay conscious and alive, another part of their brain hovers, unmoored, above the scene. "It almost felt like a movie set. You just go into this weird space where you're slightly detached from reality. It's like you're just not making any conscious decisions but watching yourself do something. I felt like I was playing out the theory of what I would do in that situation." The danger is palpable. The vehicle in which Sam crouches beside Bradley creaks and ticks like a bomb—something they choose, or are compelled, to ignore. "There was loads of smoke coming from the car. It was ticking as well. I couldn't see any flames, but something must have been on fire. I kept thinking, 'In the movies this car would explode, but that's not going to happen, that won't actually happen.' I didn't know who I was because apparently I was the type of person who would get into a burning car with a child. I didn't think I could do that."

Meanwhile, at the back of the car Nick is momentarily floored. *This isn't good*, he thinks. *This isn't good at all*. He stares at Keira, who hangs limply from her seat belt. "I was looking at a little girl who wasn't moving and wasn't responding, whose neck was at a funny angle and who was turning blue," he says. Nothing in Nick's training has prepared him for this. Every detail of the scene screams the same imperative: act now, do not delay—because if you dither, if you doubt yourself, this child is going to die.

In the slew of adrenaline, events crack into fragments. Smoke. Unresponsiveness. Someone hands Nick a mobile. A 999 dispatcher is on the line. Nick starts narrating the scene in clipped medical terms—the number of victims, the gravity of the injuries, the ominous color of deoxygenated blood. There is no crash team, no cavalry to help him, and two thoughts now hammer Nick's skull. One: *She is blue, she is suffocating before his eyes*. Two: Her cervical spine, or C-spine, looks deformed, as though it may be broken. And if indeed the child's neck is fractured, then any attempt to free her from the twisted metal could fatally sever her spinal cord. Nick possesses, in short, enough knowledge to understand that his next act—or failure to act—might kill the little girl. The thought is outrageous, enough to make a person keel. Keira's life rests entirely in his hands.

————

Forty-one years and five months earlier, on an icy evening in February 1976, Dr. James Styner, an American orthopedic surgeon and qualified pilot, encountered low cloud while flying his light aircraft, a six-seater Beechcraft Baron, across the frozen prairies of Nebraska. What happened next was both tragic and revolutionary for the practice of trauma medicine.[5]

Styner was flying his wife and four children, ages three, seven, eight, and ten, home to Lincoln, Nebraska, from a wedding in California. It was early evening and already dark when the unexpected cloud loomed. The surgeon's options were limited. A storm to the rear prevented him from turning back, and he lacked the required instrument clearance to fly safely upward through the cloud bank. The only alternative was flying lower and lower to stay beneath the encroaching cloud. Experienced pilots will tell you that the cardinal rule of low-level navigation is always to maintain an escape route. Styner had none. Nor, as his altitude dropped, did he have visual contact with the terrain beneath him. The inevitable happened. A moment of disorientation, the ground rushing upward, the smash of branches through the glass of the cockpit, the shriek of metal meeting dirt at 168 miles per hour.

Styner spent the next eight hours alone on a prairie in subzero temperatures, attempting to keep his family alive. His wife had died instantly on impact and all of his children were seriously injured. Styner himself had suffered a chest trauma and a fracture of his orbit, the bone encasing the eye. Blind in that eye, but with the help of his oldest son, he managed to pull the three unconscious younger children from the wreckage. Recognizing the dangers of hypothermia, he gathered as much clothing as possible from their suitcases and created a nest in which he placed all four children, instructing them not to move as he set off alone to find help. At 2 a.m., two travelers in a truck were startled when a screaming man, bathed in blood, staggered into the middle of the road. With a cargo of five critically injured passengers, four of them pediatric, the men drove as quickly as they dared to the nearest hospital.

This should have been the moment when the family's plight improved. Instead, the care provided at the small rural hospital would prove to be so substandard that Styner later described his family's eventual evacuation to a large urban center as "coming out of a hostile hell into civilisation."[6] Despite possessing an emergency department, the rural hospital was closed and locked overnight. There were no doctors on-site. At first, when Styner hammered on the glass to be let in, the nurse on duty refused, telling him he would have to wait for a doctor to arrive before she would admit them. When she saw the smears of blood left by Styner's palms on the glass, the nurse relented and unlocked the doors. According to Styner, however, she was visibly agitated and overwhelmed by the number of victims. Two on-call doctors, both general practitioners, finally arrived, but they, too, were disorientated and unsure how to triage the sudden influx of patients. Styner was horrified when one of the physicians—with no apparent concern for a potentially injured C-spine—lifted his semiconscious son off a gurney, causing his unsupported head to loll backward. None of the children's spines were immobilized, nor were they investigated for spinal fractures. The local medics were simply unaware such procedures were necessary.

Styner was so appalled by the chaos that he called a colleague at Lincoln General Hospital, who arranged for the family to be evacuated there by helicopter. At 8 a.m., fourteen hours after the crash,

Styner and his children arrived at Lincoln General, where a team of emergency medics and surgeons had been assembled, waiting to swoop into action. Several surgeries and much expertly choreographed critical care later, all four children survived.

In the months that followed, Styner could not stop reflecting on the perilous nature of his family's initial care. He later wrote: "When I can provide better care in the field with limited resources than my children and I received at the primary facility, there is something wrong with the system and the system has to be changed."[7] Remarkably, that is exactly what he did. Styner worked with colleagues at Lincoln General to devise a basic, logical protocol for how to manage trauma patients. Building on the work of another Lincoln physician, Steve Carveth, who had invented an algorithm called advanced cardiac life support (ACLS) for use in cardiac arrests, Styner decided to call his version advanced trauma life support (ATLS).[8]

The genius of ATLS lay in its simplicity. The protocol deployed no innovative techniques or radical management principles. Rather, Styner recognized that the fundamental problem in managing trauma was not doctors' incompetence but the lack of a systematic approach to trauma victims, plus the use of obsolete methods. What was needed was fairly simple, he wrote. There was a basic lack of consistency and they needed a way to address this. In other words, they required a method of educating physicians in how to treat trauma in a systematic manner that was applicable to all facilities across the state.

The bedrock of ATLS is the awareness that with a traumatic or violent injury, time is of the essence. ATLS is a means of ordering and prioritizing treatment in the "golden hour" immediately after a trauma. The underlying principle is simple: know what will kill the patient fastest, fix that first, and only then move on to the next thing. If a patient is bleeding profusely, for example, this may look dramatic and life-threatening, and indeed can kill. But attending to the bleeding while ignoring the fact that the patient is quietly turning blue from their crushed chest and punctured lungs will rapidly lead to their death.

With elegant simplicity, ATLS follows the structure A, B, C, D, E. Airway comes before Breathing, which comes before Circulation, which comes before Disability, which comes before Exposure. The clinician performs a rapid, urgent "primary survey" in which they must first check the patient's C-spine and airway. Only if both are intact and protected can they move on to assessing the lungs. If they judge the patient to be breathing effectively and hence capable of oxygenating their blood, they can move on to assessing how effectively that blood is circulating, and so on.

Styner summarized the power of ATLS as being "everyone involved with the trauma victim speak[ing] the same 'ATLS' language. This ability to communicate and anticipate at all levels decreases morbidity and mortality in the golden hour."[9] He tested out his new training course with some physicians in rural Nebraska in 1978. The course was a resounding success. The following year, the American College of Surgeons' Committee on Trauma adopted it nationally, with the US military swiftly following. Today, ATLS has been taught to over a million doctors in over eighty countries, revolutionizing the way acute trauma is managed worldwide.[10] It gives doctors, nurses, and paramedics a scaffold to cling on to amid the shock and disarray of a major trauma, a mantra that is drilled in so thoroughly it is never forgotten. As Styner memorably put it: "Out of the mass of the metal, the injured, the dead, ATLS was born."[11]

———

Nick Hillier stares at the little girl whose head lolls askew and whose lips are stained blue. Just over a year earlier, while still a medical student, he attended a two-day ATLS course precisely designed for situations like this, but his training has never been put to the test so exactingly. "I just thought, where do I start? What do I do? My brain clicked into what was going on here. What are the priorities and what do we need to do there and then? I thought, 'We must get her out of the car really quickly.' That was the only thing that matters."

In an ideal world, Nick knows, he would not extract Keira from the car without first immobilizing her C-spine. But reality forces his hand. She has no signs of life, neither breaths nor a heartbeat. Her lungs have ceased inflating; her blood no longer flows. Without oxygen, Nick is all too aware, the brain survives intact for roughly three minutes. If he doesn't attempt CPR immediately, Keira will not stand a chance. Together with several members of the public, he carries the child from the crumpled metal. "I was trying to hold her neck as best I could," says Nick. "We got her out and I went to the head end as soon as she was out. We moved her over onto the side of the tarmac and we were just by the roadside. One of the others was saying, 'I'm not sure if I can feel the pulse,' but I said, 'Don't bother, we need to start CPR now because there's no signs of life—let's not mess about.' I got the others doing chest compressions, taking turns and counting them out for me. Every time they got to fifteen they stopped and I gave two rescue breaths."

There is a desperate quality to the attempted resuscitation of Keira. "I remember thinking while we were doing CPR, 'Is this actually just futile?' I didn't really want to say that or go there. But in my head I was thinking, 'What are we even doing?'" Nick fears that Keira's C-spine may have been fractured or dislocated in the collision, causing her vertebrae to block her airway. His rescue breaths, instead of easily filling her lungs with air, seem to meet with disconcerting resistance.

From across the tarmac, still seated inside the ticking and smoking Vauxhall Vectra, Sam sees Nick kneeling beside the figure of a tiny girl. "I just thought, 'I am watching someone die on the ground,'" they say. "I thought she was dead. I didn't think she was coming back." Dazed, overwhelmed, still talking to Bradley, Sam dimly registers that this is not remotely what they had imagined a serious traffic accident to be like. "I remember thinking, 'It's funny how there's not that much blood.' I was thinking it would be gory, but it's not. It's that this person is the wrong color, or the wrong shape."

It takes an air ambulance thirty minutes to arrive at the scene. Eventually, Nick becomes aware of noise and commotion. "I looked around and there'd been all sorts of activity while I'd been, like, lost in this little bubble. There was a helicopter landing in the field and vehicles and flashing lights and all sorts. And these guys turned up in paramedic outfits with all sorts of boxes and stuff. The paramedic introduced himself by name. I kept saying, 'I've not got the airway, I don't have the airway.'"

When the paramedics take over the care of Bradley, Sam is at last able to leave the car. Turning to find Nick, they glimpse him squeezing a bag of saline into Keira's arm, still heavily involved in the resuscitation effort. So Sam walks alone through the twin lines of stationary traffic, numb and dazed. They observe children who have climbed out of their parents' cars and are jumping up and down, thrilled by the real-life drama of a helicopter touching down before their eyes. The children badger their parents with questions. *Mum, Dad, what does it mean? Is anybody hurt? Has someone died?* "That was really surreal," says Sam. "All these children talking excitedly and stuff. One of the parents said, 'Oh, no—that's just an ambulance to look after people.' I had to say, 'Yeah, yeah. No one's hurt.' I was pretending to these kids that everything was fine."

In the days and weeks that follow, Nick cannot stop ruminating over his actions. "I went over every little bit of it in my mind. Had I done something wrong because I hadn't made the decision soon enough to get her out of the car? I kept worrying that I had caused her a brain injury, still kind of doubting myself for ages because I hadn't been able to secure her airway and maybe caused more harm." Sam, who will go on to develop post-traumatic stress disorder (PTSD), cannot stop reliving the enormity of how they risked their life inside a burning car. Their partnership, already strained by the pressures of Nick's first year of medicine, will become increasingly brittle. "I think that that was probably the beginning of the end of our relationship," says Nick. "I felt like I'd been adequately brutalized as a junior doctor to deal with it, and Sam hadn't, and they were really traumatized and upset by the whole experience, and didn't understand how I wasn't more upset by it or more traumatized by it."

In times of crisis, of rupture, unpalatable truths can emerge. For both Nick and Sam, the collision exposes a fundamental, and irresolvable, irony about the impact of medicine on their relationship. "We'd been drifting apart that whole time because Nick was so upset by the things he saw at work and he refused to talk to me about, because he said he didn't want to share something so horrible," says Sam. "Then he later said it was all pointless because I ended up being there for the worst thing that happened. We were there on that side of the road. It was horrible because there was no crash button, no team of doctors and nurses that all run in. We were alone."

———

By late afternoon, the wreckage has been towed away. Bradley and Loanna have long since been rushed by air ambulance to the nearest major trauma center in Bristol, while Keira and William Paddon have been transported by road to North Devon District Hospital in Barnstaple, from where Paddon will be able to go home after a couple days. Nick and Sam, too shaken to drive, spend several hours at a friend's house before nervously resuming their motorbike journey home. At the scene of the crash, all that remains of the horror of the morning are hundreds of tiny shards of glass, glinting like jewels from the roadside.

Despite it all—the distress, the trauma, the disintegration of their relationship to come—Sam remains certain of one thing: "If me having PTSD was the price to pay for Keira surviving so that her family could see her again, that was worth it. So, yeah. Yes."

Max

You hold the tiny glistening body that has just emerged—blood-ied, battered, howling, everything—and the flood of love is so immense it turns all the loves you have ever known into nothing but timid rehearsals. It was like this when Paul Johnson first cradled his son Harry. And again, two years later, when Harry's brother, Max, was born. "Nothing prepares you, nothing comes close," Paul says. There's the enormity of going home from the hospital, your heart thudding as it never has before, as if trying to escape its cage of bones. The absolute dependence of this small being, curled into himself like a comma. The impulse to surrender everything—job, home, health, life—to shield this new baby from the myriad ways the world could hurt him. The knowl-edge that no matter how much you wish it otherwise, the world is a capricious place in which no one can guarantee anything. The wonder and terror, in short, of parenthood. You stare at the crumpled creature wrapped in hospital cotton and think, *If I had known in advance how much I would love him, would I have been able to go through with it at all?*

———

Seven months and twenty-two days before Loanna Ball's car col-lided with a pickup truck in Devon, another set of parents' lives were overturned. On December 9, 2016, Emma Johnson, Paul's wife, found herself sitting in the relatives' room of a pediatric intensive care unit—all pastels and reverence—as though IKEA art and lavender walls could possibly soften the blows that rained down in here. She was sitting opposite one of the hospital's most experienced pediatric cardiologists, Dr. Salem Rahouma. Between them, strategically placed, was a box of NHS tissues. A few doors away lay Max, Emma's eight-year-old son, barely conscious in an intensive care bed.

From time to time—too often in Salem's specialty—doctors are required to utter words that drop like stones upon a parent's chest, crushing air and hope from the lungs. Salem knew that what he was about to say was inconceivable. Yet he needed Emma, above all, to hear and understand him. With devastating clarity, he unveiled the statistics. The problem with Max's heart, Salem said, is a condition that has a 33 percent chance of resolving, a 33 percent chance of needing a heart transplant, and a 33 percent chance of death.

Horrifying odds, enough to render a parent dumbfounded. Emma asked Salem what the word "resolve" meant. "Obviously 'resolve' is a regular word," she says now, "but I couldn't understand it. My brain had frozen. I couldn't grasp what he was saying." Salem took a moment to arrange his words. Carefully, gently, having seen this many times before, he explained that "resolve" meant getting better. Max's chances of getting better were only one in three. Small wonder Emma's mind was in free fall.

Dilated cardiomyopathy—the condition with which Max had just been diagnosed—had emerged so insidiously that Emma and Paul scarcely noticed at first. A dry cough, mild and persistent. Yet Max had also romped and raced his way through the long summer vacation of 2016, intoxicated by six weeks off school. "He was a miniature power pack, fully charged with life," says Paul, "the type of boy who would practically jump out of bed in the morning because he was so excited about the day ahead. Every little new thing he experienced was exciting to him. He was never a sedentary child." Max's cough was eclipsed by an abundance of health. He wasn't ill; he was irrepressible.

By early autumn, though, the cough was accompanied by wheezing and moments where Max seemed to gulp for air. One evening, as Emma soaked in the bathtub, Max came in and stood on the bathroom scale. *That can't be right*, she said when he told her his weight. *You were heavier than that a year ago. Well, that's what it's saying*, Max retorted. "And because of that, I started properly looking at his body," says Emma. "When you're busy, distracted, they're all just skinny kids. But suddenly I realized I could actually see his ribs. He was really thin."

Sufficiently concerned to book an appointment with a GP, Emma and Max returned with a diagnosis of asthma and a bag of inhalers, none of which seemed to help his breathing. Repeated GP appointments generated new prescriptions for more potent inhalers and copious amounts of parental reassurance. "It wasn't that we didn't express our concerns, but we were being told, 'No, no, no, don't worry, it's just asthma.' So there was nothing on our radar, no knowledge to suggest that this was anything serious," says Emma.

During October half term, Max's behavior became more unusual. The Johnsons had driven to Cornwall for a vacation. But when Emma, Harry, and Max set off up a gentle hill to visit a castle—the kind of slope Max used to take at a sprint—he was so exhausted that he struggled to walk, begging his brother for a piggyback ride. Then, in the warm indoor swimming pool, Paul found himself frowning in confusion at the bluish tinge of his youngest son's lips. He looked more closely. "I'll never forget it. I was in the water, with Max sitting on the side of the pool. I realized I could see his heartbeat all the way down here in his abdomen. You could see it clearly beating below the ribs." But even then, alarm bells were absent. "I think I probably thought, 'That's really odd—I've never seen that before.' And if I'd seen him at the start of summer and then again in half term I'd have been like, 'My God.' But when you're with somebody every day, the change is almost hiding in plain sight."

By November, other people were starting to notice that Max was not himself. The leader of his scout pack took Emma to one side to tell her that Max had asked if he could referee a soccer match because he was too tired to sprint across the field. Then Max confided in his primary school teacher that he was sad because he wasn't able to run around like he used to. Emma felt pinned between her instinctive unease that something was profoundly wrong with her child and the repeated reassurances from those with the authority of a medical degree. "He was slowly starting to slip away from us," she says. "I knew it."

It took an independent perspective to propel her into action. Max tagged along when she visited a nail salon one day. He was making the same coughing and gasping noises that had been dismissed so many times by doctors as innocuous. The manicurist felt otherwise. She said, "Have you noticed Max is gulping air a lot?" For a moment, with startling clarity, Emma saw her son through someone else's eyes. "It was almost like I needed a third party outside the family to properly see it, to help me notice it. I suddenly had a really bad gut feeling that I had to get him to the GP straightaway, that there was something dreadfully wrong. It was a feeling of impending doom. I didn't know what it was, I had no idea it was the heart, that's for sure, but I had to get him help."

Half expecting the GP receptionist to tell her the next available appointment was in three weeks' time, Emma was simultaneously relieved and fearful when instead the receptionist took one look at Max and immediately asked a GP to see him. Still, the explanation offered was asthma. This time, though, Emma had had enough. "'Hang on a minute,' I said. 'He's losing weight, he has no energy. He is deteriorating spiritually and physically. He doesn't want to get up in the morning. His cough is like a wet carpet.'"

Finally, her concerns were heard. Auscultating Max's chest with a stethoscope, the GP found a heart murmur and agreed to refer him for a chest X-ray and cardiology appointment. But Max was teetering on the edge of an abyss. Children typically have such strong physiological reserves that they can compensate for serious illness until the eleventh hour. Though Max was still functioning, still limping his way through a day at school, his undiagnosed cardiomyopathy had acquired a deadly momentum. When the X-ray appointment came through a few days later, he could barely walk into the hospital. The radiologist agreed to show them the image. "His heart just looked massive," says Emma. "We couldn't believe it. And I remember joking to Max—'Oh well, you're just such a kind, bighearted boy,' something like that. But the radiologist was totally silent, poker-faced quiet, not betraying anything."

Too weak for school now, Max spent a day at home with Paul, coughing almost continuously. He vomited in the bathroom—not, it would turn out, the contents of his stomach but copious amounts of clear, frothy liquid from his waterlogged lungs. Paul called the emergency services and as soon as the operator heard the sound of the child's uncontrollable coughing in the background, they dispatched an ambulance. On December 8, 2016, Max arrived at Leighton General Hospital in Cheshire. Inside a dimly lit cubicle in the accident and emergency department, he lay transfixed by wires, bleeping, and digital monitoring as a junior doctor asked a series of standard questions about the history of his "asthma." Paul remembered to mention the chest X-ray from a few days earlier and the doctor disappeared to look at it.

On his return, the difference was palpable. Briskly, the doctor announced, *We're going to take you to the pediatric ward.* "He didn't give anything away, but when they drew the curtains back from the bed, I couldn't help but notice that the doctors sitting behind the desk were really staring at me," says Paul. "These were the people who had just looked at the X-ray on the computer in front of them and they knew what was coming. It was obvious to see, their eyes had just popped out of their heads." Offered no explanation for why Max was being admitted, Paul felt unable to ask for the reason. "I don't know why I just accepted it. Maybe there's this part of you that doesn't want to think the worst. You find yourself being lifted along with it. But also, you don't want to be a nuisance. You don't say, 'Hold on, stop a minute.'"

Pale and limp beneath the fluorescent strip lights, his face the color of curdled cream, Max lay and waited, eyelids flickering and closing, for the porters to take him away.

———

In the muffled darkness of the children's ward, every footstep, every sigh was magnified. A baby's cry pierced the gloom. *Shhh, shhh, it's all right, darling*, whispered its mother, her voice lilting and soft as waves on a shore. From another bed, a girl clutched her abdomen and cried out in pain. With a swish and a clink, her bedside curtain was pulled aside. Feet in socks pad-padded to and from the nurses' station, then a murmur from mother to daughter revealed that pain relief was on its way. However hard you tried not to listen, you couldn't fail to hear every word.

Paul had nothing to do but sit and wait in the shadows that magnified each sound, pain, worry, fear. Too exhausted to stay awake any longer, Max lay curled up asleep in a fetal position. "His face was turned away from me, this tiny little thing on the bed. The sense that he was so small and vulnerable was simply overwhelming. And for probably forty-five minutes, I just sat there looking at him in the darkness." Paul's right leg seemed to move with a mind of its own, tapping, jittering, as though the mounting unease he felt for his son was too volatile to contain.

At last, a doctor brushed in through the curtains and Paul stood to attention like a man condemned. The doctor was young, he recalls, with strawberry-blond hair. "I can still remember every word she said: 'We've had a look at the X-ray. This has got nothing to do with asthma. It's Max's heart, it's enlarged. We think that there is a virus attacking his heart.' And it was like *bang, bang*. It just hit me like a train, because I'm not medically trained, but if somebody says to me There's a virus attacking your heart, it's serious. I turned and looked at Max, and all of a sudden the clarity was there. It's like you're slammed into gear. Oh my God, literally, literally, literally, I just looked and thought, 'You are fighting for your life.'"

The pediatrician skillfully married candor and compassion—"It's got to be a sort of unalloyed truth; I mean, my God, how do you soften news like that?"—but Paul had prior knowledge, gleaned from science documentaries on the BBC, of precisely how gravely viruses could affect the heart. This meant the news "was like a body blow and an uppercut had landed simultaneously. Whenever I had heard of people suffering from a virus connected with the heart, the outcome had always been the same: the person had required a heart transplant. Here in the pediatric ward of Leighton General Hospital, I had the incomprehensible thought that Max might need a heart transplant. I looked at my son and I had the gut-wrenching realization that our time in this world would never be the same again."

Emma arrived, having rushed north from London, where she had spent the day running a workshop on Japanese business culture. A more senior pediatrician appeared and explained to them both that Max would need to be transferred to a specialist children's hospital. Transplant was not mentioned and Paul, wary of alarming Emma unnecessarily, felt unable to disclose his fears. He returned home to collect Harry, Max's older brother, from their neighbors' house, while Emma spent the night alongside Max in the hospital. It would prove to be the longest, loneliest night of Paul's life. "My mind was just exploding. I was terrified. It was physical as well as being psychological. A sick, lightheaded feeling. You are facing a completely altered reality, you know? What you had taken as being normal, what you had taken for granted, it's all up in the air; there's no control, nothing. There's no order, no reason to it, no comprehension. There's just a wave picking you up. I started to think about how cruel it was for Max and how, at eight years of age, nobody should be facing their own mortality. And yet this little boy was looking his death in the face. You can imagine what a swirling cosmos those thoughts were. I didn't want to get sucked into a black hole, but it was like that."

The next day, doctors in the children's ward called around to the UK's most acclaimed children's hospitals—Alder Hey in Liverpool, Great Ormond Street in London, the Royal Manchester Children's Hospital—trying in vain to find a bed for Max. Time scraped by as Emma and Paul endeavored to feign composure. When Max collapsed to the floor while attempting to walk, an emergency intensive care children's ambulance was finally summoned to rush him to Manchester. Just before Emma climbed into the back of the ambulance, the pediatric ICU doctor who would accompany Max pulled her to one side. "She said to me, 'Okay, this is just to let you know that children in Max's condition can fall off their perch very quickly. I want you to know that if we do have to stop, if something happens on the journey to Manchester, we may have to pull the ambulance over, and we will get you to sit in the passenger seat, in case we need to work on Max.' She worded it very sensitively, but the 'fall off the perch' thing was, I remember thinking, a way of saying he might die on the way."

Trying to suppress the fluttering panic in her chest, Emma sat and enfolded Max's hand in her own as rush-hour traffic brought the ambulance to a standstill. The paramedics flipped on their blue light and siren, and Emma marveled as the gridlock melted away. "It was like the parting of the waves, a miracle. I had such respect for all these drivers that were managing somehow to clear the way for us to get through." On and on they traveled along the magically emptied lanes—because every driver knows deep down that nothing more substantial than the whisper of fate keeps the people they love from the horror of such a blue-lit dash, the vehicle emblazoned with the cruelest combination of words: children's intensive care ambulance. Emma felt increasingly unhinged from reality, everything roiling inside her. Somewhere beneath that bleak subsidence—the foundations of her being knocked clean away—she clung to what the traffic signified. Because it *did* mean something. She was not alone, though adrift and falling. The drivers who cleaved this miraculous path for the ambulance to squeeze through were rallying around Max, willing him on, hoping the poor kid in the back would make it.

———

Late that afternoon, Dr. Salem Rahouma—tall, imposing, Libyan by birth—checked his watch as he grabbed a sandwich from a rucksack in his overly central-heated office. If the fragilities and breakdowns of the human form obey any kind of timetable, it's that complex hospital emergencies reliably occur at the times you are most desperate to leave work—just before 5 p.m. on a Friday, or half an hour before the end of a night shift, or in triplicate on the eve of major holidays. That evening, the pediatric cardiology department was having its annual Christmas party. Party hats and crackers in a local restaurant, the whole team attending—the consultants, the juniors, the nurses, the ward clerk, the play specialists, the physiotherapists, everyone. For Salem, lunch at five or six was not unusual, nor was the news that a pediatric intensive care ambulance was inbound, transporting a child to the unit who was so unwell he was officially "peri-arrest"—at risk of his heart ceasing to beat at any moment.

Salem had been a pediatric cardiologist for over two decades and knew from bitter experience that, in a child with dilated cardiomyopathy, cardiac arrests were invariably fatal. He could have left the new admission for one of his juniors to deal with, but what kind of consultant would that have made him? He would rather miss out on the start of the party, insisting that his juniors leave on time.

Later, Emma would have no recollection of how Max was transferred from the ambulance to intensive care. Stress had wiped her clean, erased, as though the human mind can only take so much before clamping shut like a shell. Salem, though, remembered it all. "Max was as close as a child can be to arresting," he says. "I took one look at him and saw he was thin, very thin, with a huge heart visible below his ribs. I didn't need the echo to know how serious it was. Even the first time I saw him I knew perhaps only a transplant would save him."

An echocardiogram, or "echo," is a live ultrasound scan of the heart that depicts, in real time, its size and shape, the movement of its chambers, and the acceleration of the blood as it spurts in and out. Emma's first recollection of being inside the hospital with Max was of Salem, stooped intently over her son's bare chest, wielding the echo probe with the deftness of a wizard casting spells. "I remember him so well," says Emma, "because he was the doctor who stayed, the one who stayed behind. Everyone was waiting for him at the Christmas party, but this lovely man stayed and waited so he could tell me in person what was happening to Max." It was the first of innumerable tiny acts of kindness that would define the journey to come.

In the relatives' room, Salem set about explaining, with the help of an NHS paper towel—the only writing surface at hand—how Max's heart was enlarged by a condition called dilated cardiomyopathy. He drew the four chambers, the valves, the aorta, venae cavae, and pulmonary veins and arteries, explaining how the heart had become so swollen with blood that it was too weak to pump away.

"He was humble, gentle, incredibly kind," says Emma, "but at that moment his phone rang and it was his colleagues in the pub saying, 'Where are you?' You know, 'Get your arse over here.' And he was being very sensitive because he knew I was sitting there, saying, 'I'll be there, I'll be there, I'm just with a family.' And he was very apologetic, sorry about that call, explaining it was his team waiting for him at the Christmas party, but it was all done very sensitively and I said, genuinely, 'Please don't be late for your party.'"

Then came those devastating statistics: 33 percent death, 33 percent transplant, 33 percent recovery. Salem explained there were drugs they could give to Max that would increase his heart's ability to pump—a lifeline for Emma to cling on to. "'So, there's a medicine that can help him, then?' I said. And when he said, yes, there was, I thought, 'Okay, that's positive.' I tried to be logical." Against that logic, a single refrain drummed against Emma's chest. This was her little boy's heart. It felt as if the core of him was being extinguished while she could do nothing but look on.

———

No other part of the human body comes close to matching the metaphorical richness of the human heart. Hearts sing, soar, race, burn, break, bleed, swell, hammer, and melt. They can be won or lost, cut or trampled, and hewn from oak or stone or gold. They have a temperature—warm or cold—and can be squeezed, can sink, or be thrown away. They are vessels filled not only with blood, but with our sorrows, hopes, and fears. Such is the organ's centrality to the English language that the *Oxford English Dictionary*'s definition of the word "heart" runs to a staggering fifteen thousand words.[1]

For centuries humans have regarded the heart as generating not only our pulse but our emotions and morality. The renowned Renaissance French surgeon Ambroise Paré described the heart as "the chief mansion of the Soul, the organ of vitall faculty, the beginning of life, the fountain of the vitall spirits."[2] For the ancient Egyptians in the third century BCE the heart was considered the most important of the internal organs, capable of revealing a person's true character, even after death. In the weighing ceremony at the time of a person's demise, the god Anubis—an unnerving chimera with the body of a man and the head of a jackal—would place the heart on a pair of scales.[3] If the organ was sufficiently pure to weigh less than the feather of truth, the deceased would be permitted to enter the afterlife. But if it were impure and steeped in evil deeds, the heart would sink lower than the feather and be devoured by a crocodilian monster. In ancient Greece, Aristotle asserted the heart's supremacy in all human activity. It was, he believed, the source of human intellect, pleasure, and pain, and also, crucially, the location of the soul, producing the *pneuma*, or air, that animated our spirit.[4] Even today, *heartless* means callous, cold, or cruel—a moral as well as emotional failing.

There is good reason why our ancestors located the heart at the center of human existence. Though we now understand that logic and emotion originate in the brain, through the autonomic nervous system—the unconscious neural connections between the brain and all the major organs of the body—the heart is exquisitely sensitive to both. Take, for example, our response to a mysterious noise in the house after dark. Instantly, the amygdala, the primitive part of the brain involved in processing fearful and threatening stimuli, is stimulated. The famous "fight or flight" instinct is triggered, flooding the body with the hormone adrenaline. On reaching the heart, adrenaline causes it to beat both more quickly and with greater force. Blood pressure surges, the pulse quickens, the hairs on the nape of our neck may stand on end, we breathe more rapidly and deeply, and blood is diverted from our peripheries deep into the muscles of our legs, all in preparation for fleeing danger. Every bit of this response can be sensed. The thumping palpitations of our newly primed heart may be felt so dramatically we can struggle to convey the sensation except through metaphor. My heart, we announce—a little dazed and discombobulated—it leapt right out of my chest.

Whether it is fear, joy, love, or trepidation, an emotion, in other words, is literally heartfelt. It can also be literally heart-stopping, as in the case of an extreme burst of rage or fear causing the blood pressure to surge and precipitate a cardiac arrest. It is easy, then, to see why our ancestors believed that the heart not only responded to our emotions but also gave rise to them. Today we understand that our emotions and values reside in the brain, but those symbolic connotations live on. The crux of an issue is still described as the heart of the matter. And, when trying to express our truest and most sincere selves, we do so by saying we speak from the heart, or about all that our heart desires. We confide in others our deepest secrets in clandestine heart-to-hearts.

———

It was late evening in the empty hospital atrium, the corridors deserted, the cafeteria shutters drawn. Emma arrived, small and uncertain, in the cavernous hall, gripping the crumpled paper towel in one hand. She sagged at a table, too tired to stand, waiting in the darkness for Paul to arrive. At the sound of his footsteps, she steeled herself to try and convey to her husband the enormity of everything Dr. Rahouma had told her. She would have liked to smile, but found she couldn't force her mouth to change shape. Their hands met across the tabletop—an instinctive groping for another's palm, tactility in place of words. Then Emma carefully unfolded the paper towel and began to retrace with her fingers the lines the cardiologist had drawn. *This is the mitral valve, it should close each time the heart squeezes, but the chambers are so big now that it leaks and cannot close.* He said Max's heart was like a leaky bucket. *Look, see this arrow? The blood is flowing the wrong way, it's going backward when it should be going forward.*

Emma faltered midsentence, looking at Paul. Not once before had they considered the heart in these terms—as a mechanical device designed for brute force, a workhorse whose job was simply and entirely the prosaic task of shifting blood. There was nothing remotely metaphorical about heart failure. Heart failing. Pump not pumping. Boy facing early death. It does not get starker or more literal than that. Paul began to feel overwhelmed. "That was the point where we suddenly thought, 'what in God's name have we missed?'" he says. "You know, we're sitting there asking ourselves, what have we not done? What could we have done that would have prevented this? And, of course, there was absolutely nothing, but as a parent you turn it on yourself and think, 'What did we do wrong? Why is our son here?' There were all these clues. If only we'd acted sooner, if we'd just been more assertive with the GP, if we'd just done this or we'd just done that."

As the atrium reverberated with parental guilt, it dawned on Emma and Paul that they needed to break the news to other members of their family. They reached for their phones. "I started to explain the situation to my dad," says Paul, "and I just remember saying, 'He could die.' And as I uttered those words I burst into tears. I kept saying to Dad, 'I don't want him to die, I don't want to lose him, I can't lose him.' Even though I was fully grown, you're always in some way a son, and I just wanted Dad to give parental comfort, to protect me, I suppose. You want your parent to tell you everything's going to be all right. But it wasn't. Nothing would ever be the same again."

Resuscitation

North Devon District Hospital in Barnstaple has the distinction of being the most remote hospital in mainland England. The nearest neighboring hospital is a sixty-minute drive away in the city of Exeter. Tiny in NHS terms, the North Devon has just three hundred beds. Nevertheless, its staff manages to provide round-the-clock emergency and intensive care, a stroke unit, a maternity unit, and a special-care baby unit. Unlike the vast and sprawling teaching hospitals of Britain's major cities, the North Devon is a tight-knit place. It is small enough for colleagues to quickly consider themselves friends, though that intimacy comes at a price. The hospital's far-flung location and diminutive size means the full gamut of specialties cannot be catered to. Children requiring intensive care, for example, must be dispatched to Exeter or Plymouth, each a lengthy ambulance ride away. Children are only admitted to the adult intensive care unit in Barnstaple once they have been resuscitated and stabilized, and whilst awaiting transfer to the specialist pediatric unit at Bristol.

As Hannah Greenwood prepares to start her shift on the morning of Sunday, July 30, 2017, she is relieved to note that the eight-bed adult ICU has several spare beds. Lack of capacity is a perennial NHS problem, and hospitals are invariably less fraught when not full to bursting. Hannah, thirty-two, the mother of a young girl herself, is a senior intensive care nurse in Barnstaple. She tugs on her navy-blue scrubs in the hospital changing room, pulls her dark hair back from her face into a bun, and vigorously washes her hands in the sink, sending droplets rebounding from porcelain and glass. The ritual is, perhaps, as much a preparation for work as it is a matter of erasing and remaking oneself. Survival as a staff member in an ICU environment demands a degree of shape-shifting. "In this job you have to almost go into autopilot," she says. "Today I am Nurse Hannah. I am not Mummy. I am not emotional Hannah. To do my job I have to lose my emotion, go into my nurse's role. You go through those doors and you're a different person."

Working in ICU is not for the fainthearted. By definition, the patients who require the most intensive care that modern medicine can provide tend to have catastrophic injuries or illnesses. Here lie the battered, shattered, and maimed. ICU staff will often cheerfully admit to being worriers, overanalysts, pedants, obsessives—and thankfully so. It is their ferocious attention to detail that gives critically injured patients the best .odds of survival. Although intensive care can appear bewilderingly complex—patients are often buried beneath a tangle of wires and machinery—at its core, the aims are simple. When an organ—say, the heart, liver, or brain—begins to fail, the job of the machines is to temporarily take over its role, essentially buying the body some time until that organ, hopefully, recovers. "Life support" is precisely that, the giving of temporary assistance to a body in physiological crisis in the hope that, with enough time, luck, and expertise, its broken pieces will regain their vital functions. Research shows that the more meticulous and painstaking the care, the greater a patient's chances of survival.[1]

This particular Sunday starts unremarkably. By ICU standards it is almost serene. Hannah has time to make her team a round of morning coffee. She even allows herself to think ahead briefly to dinner at home with the kids in the evening. Then, shortly after noon, a pre-alert crackles through the hospital, triggering the emergency pagers of the on-call crash team. Apologies are muttered and interactions with patients abruptly curtailed as doctors spin on their heels and dash away. Every crash call is potentially a matter of life and death, but this one is exceptional—exceptionally bad. An inbound major trauma. Someone scooped up from a roadside. A cardiac arrest. A patient too unstable to be airlifted to a major trauma center. The victim, apparently, a young child. The crash team assembles with absolute focus, its individual members pointed like blades at the task ahead, hard and cold.

"The trauma team and my team went straight down to ED [the emergency department]," says Hannah. "I was told, 'This little girl is going to be coming up to ICU, so can you get the bed space ready?'"

As Hannah sets to work preparing the child's intensive care bed, somewhere on the roads of Devon a paramedic is lurching unsteadily in the back of an ambulance, endeavoring to shock Keira's heart back to life. Chest compressions, adrenaline, more compressions, more adrenaline, while an unseen wash of grass and sky screams past. The efforts seem hopeless, doomed to fail. The paramedic knows better than anyone that the longer a heart has been in downtime, the less likely it is ever to resume its beat. Nevertheless, against the odds, multiple shocks from the defibrillator eventually manage to kick-start a pulse. It's no more than a whisper, a butterfly's breath, but there *is* a sign of life—the faintest flicker of blood in the carotid artery. After all that time without a heartbeat, Keira has been resurrected.

———

Joe Ball is several hours into his road trip. His life is in free fall, but he is yet to know it. Beneath a sky that has darkened and glowers now with the threat of rain, Joe has reached the point in his journey where the throb of the motorbike engine has become soporific. He stops for coffee and fuel at a service station some eighty miles from home. Queuing to pay, he hears his mobile ring. He digs into stiff, unyielding leathers. The screen reports eighteen missed calls, a number that's absurd except that here is the nineteenth, its number withheld, shrilly demanding to be answered. Joe frowns in confusion at the screen in his palm as the limbic part of his brain leaps ahead, drenching his body with adrenaline. Blood drains from his face, his heart begins to gallop. In a voice he hardly knows, made harsh from fear, he barks, *Who is this? What's happened? Tell me.*

Am I speaking to Joe? Joe Ball? someone replies.

No, Joe wants to say. *No, you've got the wrong guy.* Whatever words are coming next, he knows he does not want to hear them.

This is the police, Joe. I'm afraid I have some bad news. Your wife and your children have been involved in a car accident. It's serious. Your wife and son have been airlifted to Bristol for medical treatment. Your daughter has gone to Barnstaple hospital.

Joe is dumbstruck as images of devastation assail him. "I felt completely sick," he says. "I thought, perhaps they've lost limbs, broken bones, the worst. I hadn't paid for the fuel, but the cashier was taking ages, so I just threw armfuls of cash onto the counter and ran to the bike."

Wait, say the police. *Don't drive anywhere. Wait for us to come and collect you. We're coming now. Please wait.* But Joe is lost to sense and reason. "There was no way I was staying put. No chance." He is conscious of only one thing, that he must—at all costs—reach his wife and son, whose injuries are so severe they have been rushed by air ambulance to Bristol.

His fingers tremble as he struggles to tighten the strap of his helmet. He slams his foot down, and the engine roars. He is barely aware that he is racing through a deluge, an apocalyptic downpour, half blinded by a rainstorm that has burst from nowhere. In the blur of water, headlights, spray, and anguish, there is one speck of comfort to which Joe tries to cling. At least, he tells himself, Keira is safe in Barnstaple. Out of the three of them she must have escaped with minor injuries because, mercifully, unlike the others, she has not needed to be airlifted at all.

———

Hannah waits. She has checked and rechecked every inch of the bed space. In fits and starts, information trickles upward to ICU from downstairs. "We found out that Keira had gone straight into theater from Resus. She couldn't go for a scan first because her internal injuries were so severe. She needed emergency surgery," says Hannah. "For a long time, all we kept hearing was 'Oh, I don't know if she's going to make it through to you guys.' There was all that apprehension of not knowing what to expect, what would come through the doors."

In the emergency department, the handover from the paramedics to the hospital team is bleak. The time of arrival of the ambulance at the site of the crash is reported as 11:30 a.m. Keira is in cardiac arrest at this time, with junior doctor Nick Hillier and his team of volunteers performing CPR. She is deeply unconscious. Paramedics secure her airway by intubating her on the roadside—inserting a plastic tube directly into her trachea and manually ventilating her lungs with 100 percent oxygen. Next, they try to address her critically low blood pressure with bags of intraosseous saline—fluid squeezed directly through a metal cannula inserted into the tibia, the bone linking knee to ankle, since her veins have collapsed. The paramedics continue CPR in transit to Barnstaple, calling ahead to ensure that Resus has multiple bags of O-negative blood primed and ready to transfuse. ROSC—return of spontaneous circulation—is recorded as occurring at 12:25 p.m. In other words, for over an hour Keira has been in downtime, the period during which a heart fails to beat spontaneously and chest compressions alone keep the blood in circulation.

On arrival in Resus, Keira has scarcely any cardiac output. One lung has collapsed, her C-spine appears broken, and an emergency ultrasound scan shows internal bleeding in both her thorax and abdomen. As quickly as the crash team can transfuse O-negative blood, it is hemorrhaging away. Keira's only chance of survival is to go straight to theater for damage control surgery. At 1 p.m., the little girl is anesthetized. Then: press, pack, tie, cauterize. Do whatever you can to stop the bleeding as quickly as possible. This is battlefield surgery, necessarily perfunctory. Keira's emergency surgeon takes seconds to perform a midline laparotomy, a sweeping incision from the edge of the sternum to the rim of the pelvis, opening the whole of the abdominal cavity. The spleen, he sees at once, has multiple lacerations from which blood now pours. There are tears across the bowel in the duodenum, the jejunum, and the transverse colon. The liver is swollen with a huge hematoma, or blood clot, and the abdominal cavity is awash with at least half a liter of blood. The surgeon doesn't hesitate. "He did a small bowel resection for rapid control," says another emergency doctor at work that day. "Clamp, cut. Clamp, cut. You don't do definitive surgery and reconnect stuff properly because the priority is trying to stabilize the patient. You just do enough to be able to stop the bleeding and save the life. Somebody else will need to do another, definitive operation at some point—if the patient survives."

Keira leaves theater at 3:15 p.m. It has taken over two hours of high-risk trauma surgery to stabilize her sufficiently to be taken to a CT scanner. From top to toe, a radiologist scours the images for additional injuries. The CT confirms that Keira has suffered a subarachnoid hemorrhage. Her brain is swollen and there is also swelling of the soft tissues around C1 and C2, the first two vertebrae of the neck, suggesting a fracture at the critically important point at which the spinal cord meets the brain. Keira's lungs are bruised and punctured. Her left clavicle is broken. It feels merciful that she has been deeply unconscious from the moment of impact—and miraculous that she lives at all.

———

The language of medicine, though relentless in its detail, omits certain facts that Hannah Greenwood will never forget. Missing, for example, is what accompanies Keira all the way from Resus to theater, from theater to CT, and from CT into ICU. But Hannah spots it immediately, tucked for safekeeping by Keira's side. A teddy bear, soft and cuddly, with its nose embroidered in the shape of a heart, and a lilac ribbon tied in a bow around its neck. Emergency departments often keep stashes of donated teddies, widely renowned for their pediatric superpowers. Not only do the soft toys offer comfort and distraction for the hospital's youngest patients, they can also be used to demonstrate procedures, helping a child understand what a doctor or nurse intends for them. Surgeons and anesthesiologists have even been known to write up operation notes for teddies alongside their patients, ensuring that if a child leaves the theater in bandages, teddy does, too.

Hannah inhales sharply. She sees precisely what this cuddly toy represents. Amid the drama and desperation in Resus earlier, someone in the crash team has seen Keira not simply as a body, inert and unresponsive, but as a vulnerable child in need of compassion. Hannah stares at Keira's unblemished cheeks and brow, her halo of sunshine-colored hair. "Obviously we'd heard a lot about the fact that she might not make it, how she was critically injured and how much they were struggling in theater. But this beautiful little girl came through who didn't look anything like the extent of her injuries. There was no real exterior evidence of damage at all. She looked absolutely perfect. She was this little perfect girl, just lying in a bed, who was going to wake up any moment. And my first thought was 'Well, I haven't got the right child here. This can't be her.'"

Not for one moment does Hannah allow her emotions to compromise her care. "In ICU, you do whatever you have to do. As soon as you go out of those doors, it's like you almost go into a different world. When you are with a patient, you're in that sort of you-must-do-this zone; you must be on fire. You just have to go on autopilot. It's what you are trained to do. Then at some point, maybe a day or a week or two down the line, it will hit you. It hits in different ways and people respond differently. The trigger can be related, or it can be something completely random. But in the moment? You just get on with it." There is no time to waste. Despite the heroic efforts in theater, Keira's physiology has again deteriorated. The ICU team struggles to maintain almost every vital sign—heartbeat, blood pressure, and blood oxygen levels. "The day became a manic blur," says Hannah. "We were continuously doing things with the ventilator, changing the settings, because ventilation was still a huge problem. We were struggling to maintain a cardiac output. She was on huge doses of noradrenaline and adrenaline. I've never seen doses like that in a child. She was on a knife-edge."

At one point, Hannah sits with Keira, simply stroking and combing her hair. "We always try and treat our patients as human, even if they're sedated," says Hannah. "We would never do something to a patient without talking to them first. We'll say, 'Okay, I'm just going to get your hairbrush and brush your hair.' I wanted to make sure Keira was presentable to potentially see Mum and Dad. You're always aware that when any relatives come to ICU for the first time, this is going to be the image that sits in their head, that first image of their loved one asleep. So I had to try and get

Keira as presentable as possible with all these lines and tubes. I remember she had this absolutely beautiful blond, curly hair."

Information has filtered through to the ICU that Keira's father, Joe, is on his way to join her mother and younger brother in the hospitals to which they have been airlifted in Bristol. The news horrifies Hannah. She knows that if Joe is on his way to Bristol, not Barnstaple, there is a very real chance that Keira is going to die without any of her immediate family at her side. "I kept thinking, 'We need to get Joe here now because I don't know if she's going to make it.' There was this awful sense of 'Oh God, this little girl doesn't have a parent with her. She cannot die without a parent. That cannot happen.'"

All that Hannah can do now for Keira is remain hypervigilant, tweaking the dose and rate of each infusion and meticulously adjusting the ventilator settings. Every one of the child's breaths is mechanically controlled, with the ventilator pushing a mixture of air and oxygen into her lungs at precisely predetermined pressures. Without the machine at the bedside turning air into breath, Keira would already be dead.

————

Some sixty-five years earlier, another young girl lay close to death in the hospital. Twelve-year-old Vivi Ebert was struggling to breathe in Blegdam Hospital in central Copenhagen. An anesthesiologist named Bjørn Ibsen stood poised above her, instruments in hand, bathed in sweat. Not only because it was August—the height of Danish midsummer—but the procedure he was about to attempt was untried, untested, and largely based on guesswork. Ibsen was painfully aware that what he planned amounted to little more than a last-ditch medical experiment. Yet without it, his patient faced imminent and certain death. Indeed, she had been selected for precisely that reason. "A patient in a very bad condition was chosen," he would later write in a medical journal. "She was a 12-year-old girl who had paralysis of all four extremities. She had atelectasis [a collapse] of the left lung and was gasping for air and drowning in her own secretions. Her temperature was 42°C. She was cyanotic and sweating."[2]

It was 1952. Vivi was suffering from one of the most feared diseases of the early twentieth century: polio. Although improvements in sanitation and hygiene had led to the steady decline of some of the biggest killers of the 1800s such as typhoid and cholera, outbreaks of polio had grown ever more severe and widespread, and no one understood why. Polio is usually asymptomatic or causes a mild flu-like illness, but in around 1 percent of cases the virus enters the central nervous system, attacking the nerves that control the muscles.[3] Terrifyingly quickly—in a matter of hours—someone can be left immobilized from the neck down, unable to move, swallow, or breathe unaided. In his novel *Nemesis*, set in Newark in 1944, Philip Roth vividly depicts the rapidity with which polio could overwhelm its victims: "Finally the cataclysm began—the monstrous headache, the enfeebling exhaustion, the severe nausea, the raging fever, the unbearable muscle ache, followed in another forty-eight hours by the paralysis."[4]

From 1916 onward, polio outbreaks blighted American and European summers with chilling regularity. Children were particularly susceptible and there was no cure. What made the disease so terrifying for parents was that no one could predict who would walk away from an infection with a mild sore throat, and who would never walk again. Culprits blamed for spreading polio included cats, flies, possums, exhaust fumes, Italian immigrants, telephone lines, peaches, and bananas. As "polio hysteria" spread, parents kept their children behind closed doors, while councils closed swimming pools, cinemas, schools, and churches, forcing priests to broadcast their sermons on the radio. The most mundane of human interactions became laced with fear and uncertainty.[5]

Ironically, polio's resurgence was an unforeseen consequence of the recent developments in sewage and water sanitization. The virus entered the body via food or water contaminated with infected feces. But toward the end of the 1800s, the quality of the water supply in urban areas was sufficiently improved that newborn babies rarely encountered polio, while they still possessed maternal antibodies to the virus. They failed, therefore, to build up natural defenses to polio. Slowly but surely, the reduced exposure of infants to the virus weakened the population's herd immunity.[6] By the summer of 1952—the worst polio outbreak in US history—58,000 cases were reported. Of those, 3,145 died and 21,269 were left with mild to disabling paralysis.[7] The same year, according to historian David Oshinsky in his book *Polio: An American Story*, the only phenomenon Americans feared more than polio was nuclear annihilation.[8]

Vivi was admitted to Blegdam Hospital at precisely the time its doctors realized they faced a catastrophe in the making. The number of hospital admissions had exceeded anything the staff had known, yet still the patients kept coming. Around thirty to fifty patients, many of them children, were arriving every day with symptoms of bulbar polio, the most feared kind. In bulbar polio, a patient's respiratory muscles could be completely paralyzed. Then their only chance of survival was to be encased inside an "iron lung," a coffin-like box attached to a bellows that created negative pressure—a vacuum—around the body. The vacuum forced the ribs, and therefore the lungs, to expand, causing air to rush into the trachea and fill the void. Yet Blegdam possessed only one iron lung. In the first three weeks of the epidemic alone, twenty-seven of the hospital's thirty-one patients with bulbar polio died, nineteen of them within three days of admission.[9]

Barely able to breathe or swallow, saliva pooling in her unprotected lungs, Vivi was drowning before Bjørn Ibsen's eyes. The hospital's only iron lung was already in use—but Ibsen had a radical plan. Like all anesthesiologists, he prepared his patients for surgery using two groups of drugs. One class, the sedatives, rendered the patient unconscious. The other class, the muscle relaxants, caused the body to become floppy and paralyzed, enabling the surgeon to wield their scalpel unimpeded. Until the paralysis was reversed, patients in theater were unable to breathe for themselves and were attached to a rudimentary machine that squeezed air at high pressure into their lungs. Ibsen's stroke of genius was to apply this method of temporary "positive pressure ventilation" to patients paralyzed not by drugs during surgery but by polio—to Vivi, in other words.

What happened next would transform the course of modern medicine. Instead of incarcerating a patient in an iron lung, Ibsen intended to forcibly blow air into the lungs to make them expand. He aimed his scalpel at Vivi's neck, deftly creating a small incision—a tracheostomy—through which he inserted a tube into her trachea. Next, he attached a bag, itself connected to an oxygen supply, to the tube. Now every time the bag was manually squeezed, a burst of oxygen was delivered under pressure straight into Vivi's lungs. After some precarious moments, the results were spectacular. The pink flush of oxygenated blood rapidly infused Vivi's skin, and her blood pressure and heart rate stabilized.

There was just one catch. Vivi's life depended on someone at her bedside night and day, delivering every one of her breaths artificially. With up to sixty new cases of polio arriving at the hospital daily, that meant a small army of human volunteers was required. What followed was one of the most remarkable episodes in the history of healthcare. Ibsen and his team marshaled 1,500 medical and dental students from the University of Copenhagen to manually ventilate every polio patient with respiratory paralysis. For weeks and then months, in six-hour shifts, the volunteers worked around the clock, one at each patient's bedside. Thanks to their extraordinary efforts, mortality for polio patients with respiratory failure in the hospital fell from 90 percent to 31 percent.[10]

Ibsen's maverick approach demonstrated that it was possible to keep patients with respiratory paralysis alive for weeks, or even months, with nothing more technical than a pair of hands squeezing oxygen into their lungs. The discovery was a revelation. Engineers swiftly designed machines to take over the manual efforts of the medical students—precursors of the mechanical ventilators we see in ICUs today. From that point onward, anyone in respiratory failure from any cause could, in theory, be kept alive on a ventilator for as long as it took their lungs to recover.

Ibsen's achievements did not stop there. The polio patients had such complex needs that he decided to group them together in one ward for intensive management:

> All patients with respiratory problems were collected in a special department, where they were under constant observation by a team, consisting of the epidemiologist, the ear, nose and throat surgeon, and the anaesthetist, and working with help from an excellent and capable laboratory. Later on radiologists and physiotherapists also helped. . . . In order to secure continuity in treatment, conferences were held every day at which all problems were discussed. Specialists were invited to attend these conferences—physiologists, cardiologists, neurologists, &c.[11]

Unwittingly, Ibsen had just invented an intensive care unit. He had discovered that it was easier and safer to bring together critically unwell patients in one place where the doctors and nurses had expertise in severely distorted physiology, respiratory failure, and mechanical ventilation. The following year, 1953, he oversaw the setting up of Copenhagen's first dedicated ICU—with other countries swiftly following suit—earning him the soubriquet the "Father of Intensive Care."[12] At a time when the first polio vaccines had yet to be invented, he gave doctors and the public hope in the face of one of the most deadly infectious diseases of the age. Thanks to him, children all over the world lived who would otherwise have died. Vivi herself lived for another two decades after Ibsen first ventilated her. Although she remained permanently paralyzed from the neck down, requiring machinery to help her breathe, she was able to live in an apartment away from the hospital, paint with a brush held between her teeth, fall in love, get married, and cherish her life.[13]

The miraculous quality of advances in medicine is, however, famously short-lived. Since their invention in the 1950s, the use of mechanical ventilators has expanded to such a degree that anyone fortunate enough to live in a high-income country is likely to take for granted the idea that if they become sufficiently unwell from pneumonia, polio, or any other cause of respiratory failure, they will be placed on a ventilator. It took the onset of the Covid-19 pandemic in 2020 for this complacency to change. Suddenly, in countries like the US and Britain, the public woke up to the horrifying prospect of dying from a lung condition not because it was inherently untreatable, but because a lack of ventilators might force their use to be rationed. As with polio in the 1950s, the unfolding Covid-19 pandemic left a terrified world bereft of treatments, protocols, and vaccines. In early 2020, the only lifesaving tools at doctors' disposal were oxygen and the mechanical successors of Bjørn Ibsen's rudimentary ventilators.

———

By Sunday evening it is clear to all that Keira must rejoin her family. "There was never going to be, like, an optimal moment for the transfer to Bristol," Hannah Greenwood recalls. "We'd kind of done everything we could do and she wasn't going to get any better." Hannah's thirteen-hour shift has officially ended, and she is exhausted. Throughout the shift, the thought has not left her head that Keira must not die in the hands of strangers. "What really drove me was getting her to be with her parents, because that's where she needed to be. Ultimately, Keira was still alive, still with us, and that's all we could hope for. We just had to make the decision to transfer her." Hannah cannot bear to leave the unit until Keira is safely in transit. "I had to make sure she was in the ambulance, that I had done everything I possibly could. I wouldn't have been able to sleep without knowing that at least she was on the road to Bristol."

With the same tenderness and warmth she would show her own daughters, Hannah smooths Keira's hair one more time and tucks the teddy safely beneath the blankets. She checks every line, every drug, every dressing and infusion, because in intensive care you can never be too careful. At last the ambulance sets off into the night and Hannah trudges wearily toward the empty staff car park in the darkness. There will, in time, be much to feel proud of. She will recall the "absolutely phenomenal teamwork" and the way in which "every department, everyone from the porters to the cleaners to the consultants, literally the whole hospital, was carrying Keira. There were no questions, no qualms. People just said, 'Yeah, not a problem, I'll get that, I'll go there. We'll do whatever Keira needs.'" Later still, when Hannah learns about the four people whose lives will be saved thanks to the gift of Keira's transplanted organs, she will feel a sense of awe that this only happened because everyone, in multiple teams across the hospital, pulled together and did their jobs well. Most keenly felt of all, though, will be Hannah's quiet inner pride that at the end of Keira's life, far from being alone, she was cocooned in more love—from her father, mother, sisters, brother, aunties, uncles, cousins—than any of us could hope for, and that this only happened because on a quiet Sunday at the height of summer, the North Devon District Hospital did its job beautifully.

For now, Hannah is numb. "I could hardly drive I was so tired. I may have coping strategies, but that doesn't mean that I don't care. Of course you care. But you also see life for what it is, for what is precious. I got home and my daughter was asleep in bed. I didn't care that she was in bed. I opened the door and I held her tight and gave her a kiss good night—because that's what I had to do. If these kinds of events don't make you aware of how lucky you are with your own life, then there's something really amiss, isn't there?"

Crocodiles

Eight-year-old Max Johnson spent Christmas Eve 2016 fighting a losing battle to appear unconvinced of the existence of Santa. By the time the nurses handed over to their colleagues on the night shift—and every other child on the ward was sleeping peacefully—not even Max's failing heart could contain his runaway excitement.

Has he been here yet?

Max Johnson, how many times is it you've asked me that?

Yes, but has he? Has he?

No one can completely banish the rottenness for a child of having to spend Christmas away from their family in hospital, but the team on Ward 85 of the Royal Manchester Children's Hospital was giving it their valiant best. Earlier that day, the nurses had enlisted some of the younger patients to help them sprinkle a path of artificial snow along the length of the ward. A little girl had asked how they would know if Father Christmas had delivered their presents. *Because we'll find his footprints, and Rudolf's, too,* the ward sister answered. Play specialists—health workers trained in using play to help young patients adjust to their illnesses—had been hard at work with the children. Tinsel, fairy lights, and the loudest and gaudiest of homemade decorations festooned every inch of the walls. Doctors and nurses sported Christmas sweaters and flashing LED red noses. Much to the glee of every age group, the nurses had helped the children turn a pile of cardboard bedpans into reindeer displays hung on the walls. And no one quite knew who had caused the greatest stir upon their surprise visits to the ward—the Premier League soccer stars from Manchester United or the miniature ponies. "As the big day approached, it was genuinely humbling to see just how much was being done for the children to try and take their minds off the reality of their predicament in hospital," recalls Max's father.

Ward 85 is a twenty-eight-bed tertiary medical ward where children with serious cardiac, rheumatological, respiratory, and other illnesses are cared for. Its staff, states the hospital's website, "are committed to ensuring high quality care for children with complex medical needs and delivering family centred care."[1] To a twenty-first-century reader, that last phrase—"family centred care"—seems too obvious to really register. The unstinting efforts on the part of hospital staff to make children like Max feel as safe and cherished as possible are both wonderful and wholly uncontroversial. Who, today, would ever dispute the importance of parents and carers being intimately involved in a child's stay in the hospital, not least for the emotional welfare of the child? Yet if Max had been hospitalized at any time prior to the 1960s, his experience would have been painfully different and his parents would have been actively barred from his bedside.

———

Should you watch a black-and-white documentary from 1952 entitled *A Two-Year-Old Goes to Hospital*, you would receive a startling education in the unintended cruelty of the 1950s practice of isolating children from their parents while in hospital. The silent film depicts two-and-a-half-year-old Laura, an angelic toddler with huge round eyes and unruly blond curls who sits behind the metal bars of her cot, hugging a teddy to her chest with forlorn intensity.[2] Laura has been admitted to an NHS hospital for eight days to have a minor operation for an umbilical hernia. During this period, as per the draconian visiting restrictions of the 1950s, she scarcely sees her parents. Initially cheerful, she is clearly unaware her mother is going to leave her. Once alone behind bars, her face crumples and she sobs uncontrollably whenever a nurse approaches. *I want my mummy*, Laura howls. A few days into her incarceration, her anguish appears to have largely abated. She no longer cries or demands attention, but silently clings to her teddy, her expression fluctuating from anxious to haunted. Eventually, even when her mother reappears, she buries her distress, appearing blank and withdrawn.

The documentary accurately depicts hospital policy of its time. In 1949, for example, London's major hospitals almost entirely separated children from their parents.[3] Charing Cross Hospital and Guy's Hospital permitted parental visiting for only one hour a week, on a Sunday. St. Bartholomew's Hospital and Westminster Hospital were slightly more lenient, permitting twice-weekly visits of one hour. The London Hospital refused all bedside visits for children under three years old, though parents were allowed to view their child through a partition. The West London Hospital had the most oppressive policy of all, banning parental visiting altogether.

A Two-Year-Old Goes to Hospital had explosive consequences for British medical practice. Even today, the contemporary responses to the two-minute clip of the film on YouTube are extraordinary. Beneath the footage is an outpouring of comments from members of the public who recognize themselves in Laura. These commentators are adults in their seventies who, like her, endured time in the hospital as a young child in the 1940s and '50s:

This was me in 1953. I was hospitalised with pneumonia age just over 2 years and my mother only allowed to visit for 30 minutes a day. When I came out of hospital, I bit other children for a whole year until I asked my mother why she left me. She explained and the biting stopped. However the loss of trust in people, a wariness remained. I'm now 70 and still recovering from it.

I was a two-year-old in hospital in 1947. In isolation for 6 weeks with scarlet fever. At 73 I've just finished 3 years of twice weekly psychotherapy. I now have insight but not yet relief from this event in the distant past.

This was me at age five following open-heart surgery in 1955. The scars never, ever heal. It makes me weep just watching this clip. Thank God we have progressed from these dark ages.[4]

How could hospitals in the UK and US at the time have routinely inflicted such anguish and trauma on children? The restrictions arose in part from the origins of the first large urban children's hospitals in the nineteenth century. The prestigious institutions being built at this time—such as Great Ormond Street Hospital in London (founded in 1852), Royal Manchester Children's Hospital (1829), and America's Boston Children's Hospital (1869)—were independent entities predominantly funded by voluntary subscriptions from wealthy individuals.[5] They were set up specifically to provide treatment for the "deserving poor" who, unlike the pauper children of the "undeserving poor," could be spared the horrors of a workhouse infirmary provided the child's parents sought, and were granted, a subscriber's letter of recommendation.[6] Victorian values dictated other aspects of care as well, including the prevailing view among doctors and nurses that children were better off when removed to hospital and away from their impoverished, unsanitary homes and mothers who lacked the resources or character to provide the care they required.[7] Less unreasonably in the pre-antibiotic era of fatal infectious diseases such as diphtheria, polio, and measles, visiting parents were also regarded as potential vectors of infection whose presence could trigger a hospital outbreak. The exclusion of parents was therefore justified on safety grounds.

By the early twentieth century, parents, toys, pictures, and pets had largely been erased from children's wards.[8] Although such restrictions were framed as being better for children and better for parents, in truth they were also more convenient and less disruptive to the traditional working patterns of medical and nursing staff, with contemporary researchers noting the prevailing attitudes:

> Parents brought filthy germs into the wards and only upset their children, who would be crying for hours after they left, causing the nursing staff much trouble. Parents only wished to visit their children for egocentric reasons; they were being over-anxious and neurotic. The children themselves certainly did not need the visits; they quickly felt at home in the hospital. Besides, even if a child was not happy (and some doctors and nurses admitted that these children existed) it was always better to have a sad child than a dead child.[9]

In this context, the making of *A Two-Year-Old Goes to Hospital* in 1952 could be described, in twenty-first-century parlance, as an activist campaign. The driving forces behind its broadcast were the British psychiatrist and founder of attachment theory John Bowlby and the sociologist and psychoanalyst James Robertson. Both worked at London's Tavistock Clinic. Bowlby took strong exception to the behaviorist views popularized by the American psychologist John Watson who, in 1929, encapsulated his uncompromising principles of child-rearing as follows:

Treat them as though they were young adults. Never hug and kiss them, never let them sit on your lap. If you must, kiss them once on the forehead when they say goodnight. Shake hands with them in the morning . . . try it out. . . . In a week's time you will be utterly ashamed of the mawkish, sentimental way you have been handling it.[10]

In contrast, Bowlby and Robertson's research led them to believe that the abrupt separation—for whatever reason—of a young child from its parents was traumatic and could cause incalculable psychological harm. Children, they argued, needed to develop strong emotional ties with a primary caregiver, and when they lost—or believed that they had lost—those ties, the psychological impact was often devastating.

On November 28, 1952, *A Two-Year-Old Goes to Hospital* was screened before a large audience of doctors and nurses from the Section of Paediatrics of the Royal Society of Medicine in London.[11] It was met with a hostile reception. Robertson would later recall members of the audience accusing him of having "slandered paediatrics," demanding that the film should be withdrawn.[12] The film was met with such resistance from within the medical profession that when Robertson asked the BBC to show it on national television, the BBC's director general, after consulting various eminent and high-profile pediatricians, refused to do so on the grounds that it would provoke too much anxiety in parents.[13]

As a direct result of a doctor and a nurse from one small children's hospital—Amersham General in Buckinghamshire—viewing *A Two-Year-Old Goes to Hospital*, the hospital introduced a policy of open visiting, which included permitting mothers to stay overnight with their children.[14] The pace of change accelerated. In 1957, Robertson gave evidence to a parliamentary committee on the Welfare of Children in Hospital, chaired by the orthopedic surgeon Sir Harry

Platt, who concluded parents should be allowed to visit their children in hospital as often, and for as long, as possible:

> Greater attention needs to be paid to the emotional and mental needs of the child in hospital, against the background of changes in attitudes towards children, in the hospital's place in the community and in medical and surgical practice. The authority and responsibility of parents, the individuality of the child, and the importance of mitigating the effects of the break with home, should all be more fully recognised.[15]

In 1960, a small group of mothers, propelled into action by the film, formed a pressure group, Mother Care for Children in Hospital, which campaigned tirelessly to force children's hospitals to open up their visiting. The organization evolved into a powerful pressure group, England's National Association for the Welfare of Children in Hospital, with affiliate groups across the globe in Scotland, Wales, the US, Australia, New Zealand, and Europe. Over the next two decades, British society underwent a massive shift in thinking about the psychological needs of children and the consequent obligations of hospitals to fulfill these. By the 1990s, these changes had culminated in the hospital environment that Max would be lucky enough to experience, one in which parents, grandparents, sisters, brothers, cousins, teachers, toys, activities, playrooms, occupational therapists, and play specialists had all become as familiar on children's wards as they are today.[16]

———

Max's parents, Emma and Paul, were unable to sleep on Christmas Eve, despite being lucky enough to have been given parental accommodation on the hospital site. Without such rooms, in this case funded by Ronald McDonald House Charities, many parents would face the agonizing dilemma of being separated from their sick child by sometimes great distances, or of getting into insurmountable debt with sky-high hotel bills. Children's emotional needs, it seems, are indeed valued more highly today than in 1950s society—but only up to a point.

It was hot and stifling in the cramped room. Emma stared at the ceiling as sirens punctuated the night from the ambulances ferrying luckless patients to the hospital. What preyed on her mind more than anything was whether Max would be able to enjoy, however briefly, Christmas dinner away from the ward with his family. She still struggled to compute the fact that, in October, Max had been going to school, yet now his heart was so enfeebled it could barely keep him alive. His transition from an ostensibly healthy schoolboy into a critically unwell hospital inpatient had been swift and brutal. No one in the family had remotely come to terms with this. "I just wished it was me," says Emma. "I would have given anything for it to be me instead of Max."

Clair Noctor, fifty-five, a pediatric cardiac specialist nurse, met Max on the day he arrived on Ward 85. "I came in and was told that there was this eight-year-old who had an incredibly poorly functioning heart and we had no idea why. Perhaps it was genetic, perhaps infection, but he had suddenly got this hit to his heart. I remember going down to the ward and hearing screaming. Someone was trying to put a cannula into his hand. I said a brief hello to Mum and Dad, then left. Later, when he could talk, Max and I gradually began to build up a friendship."

Clair is a highly experienced pediatric nurse who originally received her specialist training at London's Great Ormond Street Hospital. As well as being responsible for more pediatric heart surgery than anywhere else in the UK, Great Ormond Street is one of the largest centers for heart transplantation in the world. In 1962, a team from the hospital developed the first-ever heart-and-lung bypass machine for children. Clair was taught by the best. "I remember Max as this very underweight, very small boy, with huge eyes and white blond hair and speakers all around his bed," she says. "He was completely obsessed with loudspeakers and technology and tried to explain all the different things that he wanted for Christmas, something about a drumbeat or boom box. I really had no idea what he was talking about."

Clair hoped to build sufficient rapport with Max and his family so that she could ease them into confronting the realities of a potential heart transplant. She knew, though, that in the short term, what would help Max the most was some structure as he languished in hospital. "You cannot normalize a child being in hospital for five weeks, let alone a year. But what you can do is help them get into a routine that gives them some structure and helps them feel secure. You know, 'You've still got to get up at breakfast time, Max. You've still got to eat a little bit, Max. You've still got to get washed and do a bit of schoolwork.' Anything to break up the monotony of things and all the uncertainty."

Since Max's arrival in Manchester, the function of his heart had been stabilized with an intravenous drug called milrinone. A so-called positive inotrope, milrinone works by increasing the force with which the heart muscle contracts. It also dilates the blood vessels in the lungs, meaning the air spaces are less congested with fluid. "It's a bit of a miracle drug," says Clair. "They can get amazingly better. Max perked up on it. He was in really good spirits by Christmas, animated, very chatty." For all the superficial improvement, Clair was under no illusions that Max was not, in all likelihood, going to require a heart transplant. Nor was his consultant cardiologist, Dr. Salem Rahouma: "I remember the severity of Max's condition. It is rare to see a cardiomyopathy so severe. I knew he could die at any time. He was at very high risk of a cardiac arrhythmia and a cardiac arrest. And we knew that if he arrested, there was almost zero chance that CPR could get him back."

Despite—or perhaps because of—the odds faced by so many of the children on their ward, that night the nurses pulled out all the stops to create something of the magic of Christmas. At midnight, having checked one final time that even Max was properly asleep, a nurse on Ward 85 picked up the phone to summon the on-call junior doctor. As she waited for him to call her back, she silently surveyed the children in their beds, from the ends of which dangled the hospital version of a Christmas stocking—an empty NHS pillowcase. The phone on the nurses' station shrilled. *It's time*, she murmured into the receiver with all the gravity of a jewel thief masterminding a heist. Five minutes later, the doctor appeared. Sack in hand, he permitted the nurses to primp his red robes and polyester beard before dutifully setting off along the trail of fake snow, pausing at each sleeping child's bed to stuff their pillow with presents donated by the hospital charity. The nurses clinked their glasses and whispered, *Happy Christmas*. It was ludicrous, absurd, and beautiful.

The next morning, Paul and Emma sat on tenterhooks at Max's side, waiting for the arrival of the doctors on their Christmas morning ward round. Family friends had brought Max's older brother, Harry, to the parents' accommodation block and were busy preparing a Christmas feast for them all. The whole family was desperate for Max to be permitted to leave the ward. "I don't think we really appreciated it at the time, but it was a real judgment on the part of the doctors," says Paul. "I remember the consultant cardiologist coming in and looking at his chart, speaking to others, and her cogs clearly cogitating. It was a real risk, it was absolutely a risk. You could almost tell that the better judgment would have been to say to us, 'Sorry, but Max is going to have to stay here.'" Instead, the doctors conferred. They were aware that if they disconnected Max from his intravenous milrinone, the half-life of the drug ought to allow it to continue to support Max's heart for the next couple of hours, albeit with dwindling force. On the other hand, his heart depended almost entirely on the milrinone to continue beating. If the infusion was stopped, at some point the diluted remnants of the drug in Max's bloodstream would be insufficient to sustain an effective heartbeat. Then, the worst-case—and entirely plausible—scenario would be a cardiac arrest from which Max would not recover. "They weighed it up," says Paul, "and in the end there was that compassion. Max needed this. It was Christmas Day. They said, 'Okay, you can go and have a couple of hours with your family. Let's disconnect the battery for two hours. Go and have some fun.'" With bandages around his wrists to protect his cannulas, Max was escorted off the ward by his parents in a wheelchair. No one knew it yet, but this would be the last time that he would leave hospital without a nurse by his side for the next seven months.

Christmas Day was not what Paul and Emma had hoped for. Although delighted to have escaped the ward, Max was wan and exhausted. Too tired to attempt to chew Christmas turkey, he grimaced as Emma tried to coax him into trying a few bites of salmon. "He just couldn't eat, he was too weak," says Paul. "Towards the end of the meal we could see him visibly flagging. We took him in his wheelchair to open his presents and he did seem genuinely distracted by the excitement of his new set of Bose speakers, but then Emma and I looked at each other and said, right, we'd need to get him back now. He was only with us for about ninety minutes—hardly any time—but it was the last time he was ever disconnected from his lines until after his transplant. The last time he was free to turn three hundred and sixty degrees."

From Christmas Day onward, the decline was precipitous. Increasingly frequently, Max became quiet and still, lying on his side in order to breathe. His waterlogged lungs, bloated with the fluid that his heart could no longer pump away, sometimes caused him to feel so nauseous he would end up vomiting. "You could see his breathing become shallow and fast," says Paul, "and he'd become so breathless he'd struggle to get enough oxygen into his system and start 'gulping' for air. It was awful to watch." One day, Paul noticed a bump in the middle of Max's chest, where his sternum had begun to protrude outward. When the doctors explained that the deformity was being caused by how grossly overstretched Max's heart had become, Paul grew silent as the statement landed. Max's body, fighting for oxygen, was flogging his heart with relentless adrenaline, driving the organ to beat and beat until the culmination of that percussive labor was enough to misshape bone. It was so unnatural, so obviously wrong, that Paul had to fight to maintain his composure. "You hold on to any hope you can at times like this and I guess that is why doctors are so careful with their use of language. In the early days, Max's heart function had improved slightly, but let's put this into perspective. It had gone from truly awful to just really awful. And now it was even worse." Paul could not stop ruminating on the fate of thirds: 33 percent will survive, 33 percent will need a transplant, 33 percent will die.

When Clair Noctor returned from leave a few days after Christmas, she took one look at Max and felt a sense of foreboding. "He was very quiet with really dark shadows underneath his eyes. He looked terrible. And his breathing was very quick, but very shallow. He just didn't have a spark anymore; he'd lost what he used to have before Christmas. I heard from the junior doctors that the team had tried to get him off intravenous milrinone and onto tablets, but he couldn't cope with it and now he was getting worse every day." The strain on Emma and Paul was palpable. Clair was concerned for Paul in particular. "Emma was the strong one. She cried and was very open with her emotions, but she also managed to listen and take everything in and step up when she needed to. Paul is a big man, very tall, towering over you, but you could see him literally crumbling physically. He was collapsing into himself. It was too much for him."

Not only were Emma and Paul struggling to come to terms with the severity of Max's illness, they were also worrying about its impact on his brother. Clair made a point of trying to support Harry, who rarely spoke in the hospital, but listened to every word that the adults uttered. "One day I said to him, 'Fancy a hot chocolate?' and his face lit up. I asked Mum and Dad if it was okay to take him to the café, and their shoulders dropped with relief, you know, because what they were going through was horrific. For any parents of a very sick child, they are having to learn all the jargon, everything about what's going on. It's exhausting." To begin with, Harry sat opposite Clair with his face turned down, stirring his hot chocolate and saying very little. Bit by bit, he began to unburden himself. "'I know they cry,' he told me," says Clair. "'They don't want me to know that they cry, but I know that they cry.' And I said, 'How does that make you feel? Does it upset you?' And he was like, 'Yeah, but don't tell them.' I said, 'Okay,' but I knew that I couldn't just let this go, and so later I had a word with Paul. I said to him, 'It was great talking to Harry and, you know, he's got his head screwed on. He knows how upset you are and he's worried.'"

There was very little, in fact, that Harry hadn't already worked out for himself. Over the course of several hot chocolates with Clair, he revealed that he knew Max's heart was not going to improve. He also knew that somebody else would have to die for Max to get better, and that this was sad, but at the same time he didn't want Max to die. "Harry was very mature for his age," says Clair, "but he was still a little boy and he'd only just started senior school. He shouldn't have had those worries. Nobody should have those worries."

By now, Max's team was in daily contact with the pediatric cardiologists at the Freeman Hospital in Newcastle, hoping he could be imminently transferred there. The Freeman, a specialist referral center built in 1977 for patients living in the northeast of England, has an international reputation as a center of excellence for cardiothoracic surgery. The Freeman had over thirty years' experience of transplanting hearts, lungs, livers, kidneys, and pancreases, and had performed the UK's first successful heart transplant in a baby in 1987.[17] This was followed by the first successful single lung transplant in Europe, and then, in 1990, the first successful double lung transplant in Europe. To date, the center has transplanted over eight hundred hearts and over six hundred lungs or lungs and hearts combined.[18] With Max now deteriorating on a daily basis—and drawing perilously close to needing the maximum possible dose of milrinone—an urgent transfer to the Freeman was imperative.

With years of experience talking to families about heart transplants, Clair introduced the topic with tact and discretion. "I think you get a clue from parents when they're ready to start a conversation. Sometimes they just want little snippets, you know? It's best to listen and just let them speak, trying to gain a bit of information from them that you can build on. You work up to the transplant, based on how much they know already, and how much more they want." For Paul and Emma, this was exactly the right approach. "Clair did it brilliantly," recalls Paul. "Without hitting us between the eyes, she introduced it almost by osmosis. It dawned on us gradually that Max was going to need a transplant. Clair and everyone else were preparing us for some big news without us even noticing, easing us towards the realization that Max's heart was beyond repair and no longer fit for purpose. Max was going to need a new heart."

With Emma and Paul, Clair was able to use sensitive language, silence, and inference in a way that allowed them to draw the conclusion for themselves. But with Max, who had only just turned nine, a different approach was needed. Together, Clair and Emma plotted out how best to break the news. "We agreed on a sort of strategy of how we were going to say he was going to Newcastle just for a heart transplant assessment, but that there was a good chance he might end up needing a new heart," says Emma. "We knew this was big news for a child, and it was. I remember Max going very quiet. Then, after a pause, he just said, 'Oh, right.' It was obviously a disappointment to him, but he didn't seem too upset. He wasn't crying or anything. In fact, Claire and I said afterwards, 'Well, that seemed to go quite well.' He really did seem to be okay about it and I felt like it had been pretty painless."

In fact, as is often the case with children in hospital, Max's silence masked a tumult of emotion. Several hours later, at around 8 p.m., Paul, who was back at home in Cheshire with Harry, received a text message from Max. Only two words in length, but with the force of a thunderclap, it read: *I'm fucked.* The language, the sentiment, the harshness, the anger—all of it took Paul's breath away. This was not his son, this was unrecognizable. The shock Paul experienced was savage, physical, a rush of pain and bile. "I felt sick to the pit of my stomach. If Max gave up, I honestly thought the situation would become hopeless. I could feel the air being sucked out of me. I felt the very real sensation of loss, there and then. I saw Max not making it, his giving up, signing and sealing his fate. That oppressive, suffocating feeling of bereavement, that you will never see that person in front of you again."

Paul picked up the phone. On the other end of the line, remote, disembodied, was his son in panic and incoherence. "I don't want to do it, Dad. I don't want it. I don't want another heart." Paul felt himself floundering. "How did I begin to soothe a child faced with such a seemingly abstract concept? How could a child who has only just turned nine be expected to react with calm reason?" He attempted to provide solace, a father's reassurance, while crippled with guilt that he could neither take Max's place nor save him from his suffering.

An hour later, Max called back.

Hi, Dad.

Hello love, are you okay?

Yeah, I'm fine. Sorry about earlier. Dad, if I need to have a new heart, I'm fine with that. Anyway, this one of mine is no good. I feel sorry for it, but it's no good. I'm fine with having a new heart.

Paul's face was wet with tears. "An adult could have been smashed by the news, but here was Max trying to bounce back for my sake. He hadn't appreciated the gravity of how ill he was before. I think it had all just sunk in and he was very, very afraid, but he was trying his hardest to be brave."

———

Max was wise to recoil instinctively from the prospect of a heart transplant—once, the medical profession did, too. The historical reluctance of surgeons to tamper with the heart stemmed in part from the awe with which the organ was regarded above all others. In the first century CE, for example, Pliny the Elder described the heart as "the primary source and origin of life," adding, perhaps self-evidently, that "when injured it produces instant death."[19] Galen, the most celebrated surgeon of ancient Europe and physician to the Roman emperor Marcus Aurelius, noted that the fatal effect in gladiators of wounds to the heart was invariably instantaneous, adding weight to the notion that the heart was inviolable. He also believed that the heart's left ventricle was where "vital spirits" were added to the blood, generating the heat and life with which it then circulated through the body.[20] Revered as sacrosanct, freighted with mystery, exalted as the repository of the human soul, the heart was where God breathed life and sanctity into human flesh, infusing us with everything that sets us apart from mere animals. Daring to carve into all that was, for much of human history, tantamount to desecration.

The first barrier to the endeavor of transplanting hearts was, then, psychological. A surgeon had to find within himself—and, until the second half of the twentieth century, surgeons *were* almost universally men[21]—the mettle to overcome the conviction that he was committing a kind of medical apostasy. That wasn't all. Imagine for a moment having the hubris to take your scalpel to an organ that not only houses the human soul but which beats, pulsates, contracts, and quivers—a relentlessly moving target. Small wonder that wounds to the heart were considered beyond the realm of a doctor's care—that cardiac surgery was essentially impossible. The retired emeritus professor of surgery at the University of London Harold Ellis notes that although the advent of anesthesia and of antiseptic surgery in the nineteenth century led to an explosion in surgery of the abdominal cavity, the chest, the skull, and the limbs, nevertheless "the heart was considered by the surgical fraternity to be the 'no-go' area of the body."[22] In 1883, for example, Theodor Billroth, professor of surgery in Vienna and revered as a pioneer of modern surgery, wrote unequivocally that "the surgeon who would attempt to suture a wound of the heart should lose the respect of his colleagues." A few years later, the American surgeon Charles Elsberg described the technicalities of why he and his colleagues baulked at operating on a beating heart:

> We must remember that we have to deal with an organ of first importance which is in constant motion, and which, moreover, was believed to be very sensitive to the smallest mechanical insult or injury. It was feared that during the slightest manipulation the heart might suddenly stop, that the mere passage of a needle might be followed by the direst results.[23]

As the twentieth century beckoned, operating on the heart remained taboo. Although surgery was now taking place on almost every other part of the human body, including the brain, if you presumed to slice into the heart, you faced potential opprobrium from your peers. Yet nothing provokes medical innovation quite like desperation. In the last few years of the nineteenth century, case reports began to appear in the medical literature of last-ditch salvage surgeries attempted on the human heart. One such operation took place in the early hours of September 4, 1896, in the National Hospital in Oslo, Norway. A young man age twenty-four was found lying in a pool of blood, having been stabbed in the chest. When the surgeon on duty, Axel Cappelen, examined the patient, he found he was unconscious with inaudible breath sounds and a barely palpable pulse.[24] There was really nothing to lose. Cappelen anesthetized the patient with chloroform and proceeded to resect the third and fourth left ribs to better visualize the heart. He saw that blood was filling the pericardial sac surrounding the heart, preventing it from beating, a phenomenon known as cardiac tamponade. Once Cappelen cleared the blood away, he was able to glimpse its source, a stab wound in the heart's left ventricle. The only way to repair the wound was to time each of his stitches with the heartbeat. An editorial in the *Journal of the American Medical Association* (*JAMA*) recounts what happened next:

> The wound was sutured and an artery tied, when the bleeding ceased. The account of the operation states that the suturing was rendered extremely difficult by the rhythmic movements of the lung, which covered the field of operating and obscured it, and by the contractions of the heart, which however were quiet and regular. The suturing was accomplished by bringing the needle

half way through a contraction, then dropping it, and after a second contraction bringing it completely through.[25]

Cappelen had just become one of the first people in the world to perform open-heart surgery. His patient survived and went on to live for another two days. A postmortem revealed pus in the pericardium, suggesting that the patient had died not from bleeding but from infection. *JAMA* reacted bullishly, noting that contrary to received wisdom about the fragile sensitivity of the heart:

The heart is an organ that sometimes tolerates foreign bodies very well. . . . Among foreign bodies found in this organ besides bullets and needles, which are the most common, are splinters of wood, fish bones etc. Even the ubiquitous hat pin has been discovered. Bullets have been found encapsulated in the heart for many years; in the right ventricle for six years; in the wall of the ventricle for twenty years; and for no less than fifty years in the pericardial sac. It must be observed in passing, however, that these cases refer to the old fashioned round balls; few conical balls will be stopped by the heart, and still fewer, if any, of the most recent projectiles of small caliber and extreme penetration.[26]

The *JAMA* editorial points out that cardiac wounds were not, in fact, inevitably fatal, citing various cases of patients surviving being shot and stabbed through the heart. It concludes prophetically: "In view of the foregoing facts, the opinion seems warranted that 'the citadel of life' itself will no longer be exempt from the incursions of the surgeons."[27]

Such surgical incursions did indeed continue apace as surgeons learned to overcome their qualms and treat the heart as if it were just another ordinary part of the body, albeit one with the unique technical challenges of perpetual motion, as it trembled and heaved beneath the theater lights. But these early beating-heart surgeries were desperate, experimental affairs, occurring most commonly in the context of battlefield injuries, when the only alternative to surgery was certain death. Case reports describing these snatch-and-grab surgeries make for lurid reading. There are "fountains of blood," "lakes of blood," surgeons operating in a "mass of bloody foam," blood spurting in great arcs into the air, and blood drenching entire operating theaters, as all the while surgeons rummage around within open chests, trying to hold their nerve while being blinded by gore.[28] In his history of cardiac surgery, *The Matter of the Heart*, Thomas Morris memorably describes the pioneering surgeries of Dwight Harken, for example, a young military surgeon from Iowa who, during the Second World War, removed bullets and shell fragments from the chests of 134 soldiers without experiencing a single fatality. "Sometimes when he cut into the heart the resulting jet of blood entirely obscured his view, and he was forced to fish around blindly for the metallic fragment in a churning scarlet sea."[29]

By the end of the Second World War, surgeons knew that it was possible to hold, manipulate, and repair the heart in precisely the same way they would any other part of the human anatomy. But for their patients to survive the experience, the heart had to keep on doing its job throughout the surgery, laboriously pumping five liters of blood through the body every minute. In the 1940s, then, the notion that you could sever a heart from its moorings in the chest, lift it up and out of its cradle of ribs, bear it in your hands to another human being lying opened like a book upon the operating table, and suture it into a new home—that was the stuff of science fiction. In 2017, Max Johnson may not have understood exactly *why* he found being told he might need a new heart so terrifying, but which of us would not have felt the same? Can anyone truly contemplate the idea of their own ransacked chest with equanimity? Even Christiaan Barnard, who in 1967 would win worldwide fame by becoming the first surgeon in the world to transplant a human heart, recognized that feeling. *Time* magazine's coverage of the historic feat captures something of the horror Max must have endured through its depiction of the ethical dilemmas faced by this new breed of surgeons who dared to dream of excising living people's hearts in order, paradoxically, to keep them alive:

Obviously [the recipient] is close to death, or such drastic surgery would not be contemplated. Yet his own heart must be cut out, which is tantamount to killing him, while he still retains vitality enough to withstand the most draconian of operations. If the transplant should fail, he will certainly die. Thus the surgeons will, in effect, have killed him (as they might in any major operation), no matter how lofty their motive in trying to prolong his life and make it more satisfying.[30]

In his autobiography, *One Life*, published in 1969, Barnard describes in even starker terms how daunting such surgery must be for patients, pinned as they are in the terrifying space between certain death without a transplant and potential death with one: "For a dying man, it is not a difficult decision [to accept a heart transplant] because he knows he is at the end. If a lion chases you to the bank of a river filled with crocodiles, you will leap into the water convinced you have a chance to swim to the other side. But you would never accept such odds if there were no lion."[31]

At nine years old, alone in the hospital, Max was trapped between lions and crocodiles, trying to protect his mum and dad by appearing to be brave.

Limbo

By the time Joe Ball's motorbike screeches into Bristol, his family, in every sense, has been shattered. It is Sunday afternoon. To the north of the city in Southmead Hospital, Joe's wife, Loanna, is barely conscious in intensive care, with multiple fractures of her arm, hand, foot, and ankle. Farther north, in the Bristol Royal Hospital for Children, seven-year-old Bradley is still losing blood from a ruptured spleen and needs immediate surgery. Back in the family's hometown of Barnstaple, a surgical team is struggling to keep Keira alive.

Joe is being wrenched in three different directions at once. Clumsy and dazed beneath sodden leather, he is led first through the corridors of Loanna's hospital, then through those of Bradley's, guided by nurses he will never recall and whose words of comfort will be forever forgotten. In the immediate aftermath of a trauma, NHS staff knows to expect stupefaction. Explanations are clear, concise, and repeated often, on the assumption that nothing will stick. In Joe's case, one thing cuts through. He knows—indeed, it is the only thing that makes a shred of sense to him—that his family cannot remain splintered. They have to be brought back together. For Loanna, this is easily achieved. She can be transferred across the city by ambulance from Southmead to the Bristol Royal Infirmary, adjacent to the Royal Hospital for Children, where Bradley is currently undergoing emergency surgery. But for Keira, the three-hour ambulance journey from Barnstaple could be fatal. Joe is undeterred. He insists his youngest daughter must be with her family in Bristol. And to the legitimate concerns that Keira could die in transit, there is one irrefutable rejoinder, the sentiment shared by her nurse Hannah Greenwood: But what if Keira dies alone in a hospital a hundred miles from either parent? In what sense could that be better? Conversations fly back and forth between the intensive care teams in Barnstaple and Bristol. Finally, at ten o'clock that night, a Pediatric Intensive Care Unit retrieval team safely delivers Keira by ambulance, on a ventilator, to Bristol.

Even before she arrives in the children's hospital, the PICU team explains to Joe that his daughter's injuries are so catastrophic she is unlikely to survive. One of the consultants, Dr. Alvin Schadenberg, recalls Joe's singular isolation: "I can still remember how awful it was that there was no one there to support him apart from us on the unit. There were no other family members and Loanna was in intensive care. Normally you'd have two parents supporting each other, but not in this case. Joe was just doing such an amazing job in that awful situation. I take my hat off to him because he had to find such strength." For Joe, subsequent events that night are less a blur than a nothingness. There are visits from the police and the pediatric neurosurgeons, more scans, more procedures, more painstaking titration of the drugs and infusions that enable his daughter's heart to keep beating. All is lost to the shell-shocked man who has nothing to hold on to save for the fact that his family has been reunited and that the horror of this night must eventually end.

———

The most important scan of the night, a CT angiogram (CTA) of Keira's brain, takes place at 2:31 a.m. precisely, on Monday, July 31. Already the PICU team fears the worst. They know that Keira's level of consciousness on the Glasgow Coma Scale (GCS) registers only a 3. Developed half a decade ago by two neurosurgeons in Glasgow, the scale is a clinical tool used to assess and calculate the nebulous matter of a patient's conscious level with as much objectivity as possible.[1] A person's GCS ranges from 3 to 15, with points being given for how vigorously a patient responds to a human voice, to being touched, and to the stimulus of pain. A fully conscious individual effortlessly scores the full GCS 15, whereas, at the opposite end of the scale, Keira's GCS of 3 means she makes no response whatsoever to voice, touch, or pain. She is no more capable of interaction with the world than is her image, captured mid-smile, beaming out from the screen of Joe's phone.

That night, in fact, everything points to Keira being brain dead. Not only is she as deeply unconscious as it is possible to be, but the PICU team knows she received over forty minutes of roadside CPR before the paramedics successfully resuscitated her heart. They are also aware that no matter how expertly CPR is performed, it is crude, rudimentary, and cannot come close to achieving the propulsive power of the human heart. CPR provides only 10 to 30 percent of normal blood flow to the heart and 30 to 40 percent of normal blood flow to the brain, even when delivered according to the guidelines.[2] This means that the longer a person experiences cardiac arrest, the greater the chances that the tissues of the brain—being exquisitely sensitive to, and hungry for, oxygen—will suffer hypoxic damage. Worse, a damaged brain tends to swell, causing a surge in pressure within the closed box of the skull. Raised intracranial pressure compresses the blood vessels, depriving the brain of even more oxygen. It is a vicious circle that culminates in brain death.[3] Already Keira's intracranial pressure is as high as the PICU team has ever seen, the most ominous prognostic factor of all.

The aim of the CT angiogram is to try to visualize the extent to which blood still circulates through Keira's brain.[4] The scan is taken immediately after a radiosensitive dye is injected into a vein in her arm. Whichever vessels contain flowing blood will now light up as the dye rushes past. As a depiction of the intricacy of the human body, a CTA of a healthy brain is hard to match. At first glance, set against the deep slate gray of normal brain tissue, the major blood vessels appear to be a furious jumble of bright white scribbles, as though a toddler has overdosed on too many sweets and gleefully taken to a blackboard with chalk. But encrypted within the fine tendrils and whorls of the digitized image is an ingenious feature. A ring of large arteries encircles the base of the brain, into which blood flows from both the front and the back of the body, via the carotid and vertebral arteries. All around the ring, multiple pairs of additional arteries branch off like spokes on a wheel, delivering blood to the brain in every direction at once. This is the famous circle of Willis, named after the seventeenth-century physician Thomas Willis, who studied medicine during the English Civil War and was the first person to use the term "neurology" in print.[5]

A celebrated neuroanatomist, Willis conducted some of his meticulous dissections of the brain and spinal cord with the assistance of such luminaries as the philosopher John Locke and the architect Christopher Wren.[6] His eponymous circle revealed how assiduously the brain protects itself against its gravest threat, being deprived of oxygen. The circle ensures that blood from any part of the brain can, in theory, reach any other part. Should a blockage in one artery disrupt the flow of blood to a particular portion of brain tissue, blood can flow forward or backward around the circle, enabling another artery to compensate. The only circumstances in which the circle breaks down are when too many vessels are simultaneously damaged—or when the intracranial pressure is so high that the compression of veins and arteries is ubiquitous.

Hunched over a screen in semidarkness, a radiologist scrutinizes the terrain of Keira's scan. Her eyes roam systematically across slices of matter, from plane to plane—sagittal, axial, coronal, oblique—

searching for the glimmers and helices and halos of light whose presence would spell hope for the child in the scanner. She is practicing, in essence, mortal cartography. Any hint of incandescence would mean flowing blood, flowing oxygen: the potential for life. But death reveals itself with flat-black finality. The radiologist traverses the frontal, parietal, temporal, and occipital lobes, then the cerebellum, the pons, the medulla oblongata, yet the darkness is absolute. At 3 a.m. she picks up the phone. It is the result Keira's doctors both feared and expected. The scan is unequivocal. All mental activity in her brain has ceased.

At half past seven on Monday morning, the PICU handover begins. Fueled by coffee, staff from the night and day shifts converge, the weariest of them propped against walls or slumped at a tabletop, eyes too bright with the excessive fatigue that comes from twelve hours straight of intensive care. Each child in the PICU is discussed in turn—their current state, any overnight events of significance, key issues for the day team to be aware of. The language is percussive—the full-tilt clatter of jargon and acronyms deployed by medics to transmit maximum information with minimum ambiguity and in the fewest seconds possible. Impenetrable to outsiders, this arcane code of PEEPs and MAPs, ET tubes and hemofilters, ECMO, apnea, FiO_2, and vasopressors has as its aim the simplest of imperatives: How do we act in this child's best interests? Can our actions enable them to stay alive?

In Keira's case, the answers are clear. Jemma Evans, one of two PICU nurses assigned to spend the next twelve hours caring for Keira, recalls: "We knew by that point that she wasn't going to make it, and that everything was complicated by the fact that her mum had been involved in the accident, so Joe was alone. The team had spent the night just trying to keep Keira as stable as possible while he tried to process what had happened. My job that day was to continue to keep her stable and let her family have as much time as they could with her, explaining what we were doing and why." A crucial decision is made during the handover. In the light of the overnight findings, everyone agrees that the day team, led by Dr. Alvin Schadenberg, should turn off Keira's sedation. It is an act that will not alter her prognosis, appearance, or care in any way—yet its significance, in due course, will be immense.

The unit contains a side room that is typically reserved for children whose injuries are likely to be terminal. Though small and dark, with neither windows nor natural light, the room grants families a degree of privacy at a time of crisis that the open-plan ward can never match. "It can feel calm, almost cozy, but because there's no window you don't see any of the outside world. It can be quite isolating in there, too," says Jemma. Inside the room, with her father dozing close beside her, Keira lies inert on her back, bathed in the half-light. Her eyes are closed; she could be sleeping. A white sheet is tucked under her chin and the elevation of the fabric with each slow breath is so slight as to be barely perceptible. With her flushed cheeks, smooth skin, and hair cascading in golden waves, she is more than merely beautiful. Radiant with the promise and potential of youth, Keira is luminous.

The machinery that surrounds the bed has an auditory signature all of its own. The multiple infusions of fluids and drugs that drip directly into Keira's jugular vein are driven by motors that issue a faint background hum, against which the sighs of her pneumatic mattress can be heard. The mechanical ventilator labors audibly to deliver each of her breaths, its components rumbling and creaking. Jemma scans the vital signs displayed on a monitor above Keira's head, digits that flicker and glow in the gloom. Blood pressure, stable. Oxygen saturations, stable. Heart rate, neither too quick nor too slow, but exactly as it should be in a nine-year-old girl. In cardiovascular terms, the fusion of pharmacology and engineering that holds Keira in this limbo between life and death is working exactly as intended.

Jemma's eyes linger on the trace of Keira's heart, a jagged range of peaks and troughs generated from multiple electrodes attached to her chest. The electrocardiogram, or ECG, depicts the electrical wave that starts spontaneously in the heart's own pacemaker—the sinoatrial node—then spreads outward and downward across the whole of the heart muscle, triggering each heartbeat. Encrypted within the digital trace is precise information about the size, shape, rhythm, oxygenation, and conduction system of the heart. It takes years for medical students and young doctors to read an ECG with finesse, and some of them, cardiologists like to grumble, never convincingly manage it. In Keira's case, the form of the ECG appears flawless. It suggests that perhaps—despite the cardiac arrest, the lengthy downtime, the major hemorrhage, the desperate surgery—this knotted fist of valve and muscle is somehow pumping with aplomb. A hardy heart, a mighty heart, a frankly inconceivable heart, if indeed it has truly survived the last twenty-four hours unscathed.

Overnight, the team has been candid. Yet the words they have deployed with Joe—*coma, very serious, we don't think she can survive this*—are starkly at odds with the visual scene. "I sat next to her that morning and cuddled her and held her hand. She looked so perfect, not broken at all. She looked like she was sleeping. I thought she was going to be all right," says Joe. The Keira he knows loves ponies, Pokémon, wearing her pink fluffy onesie, sausages, and anything orange. She longs to visit America and to work with animals. She dreams of living one day with her big sisters, Katelyn and Keely, and she will be the sensible one, cooking them meals when they stagger home from a night on the town, in need of a fry-up. Joe can feel the tremble of her pulse beneath the tips of his fingers, the warmth of her palm, the softness of her breath, and he thinks to himself, *But how can this be true, be real, if my little girl, my sleeping beauty, is not about to open her eyes?*

———————

Almost exactly a century before Joe struggled to make sense of his daughter's plight, the First World War poet Wilfred Owen wrestled with the proximity of life to death on the blood-soaked battlefields of northern France. Owen published only five poems in his lifetime. One of them, entitled "Futility," contains perhaps the most poignant description ever written of the strange hinterland a person occupies immediately after they have died. Owen contemplates its enormity as he describes a soldier, recently killed, who looks so alive to him that he cannot believe the warmth of the sun will not wake him:

> Think how it wakes the seeds—
> Woke once the clays of a cold star.
> Are limbs, so dear-achieved, are sides
> Full-nerved, still warm, too hard to stir?[7]

Those moments can be disarming, paradoxical, and deeply unnerving, even for seasoned doctors. The deceased—if briefly—remains warm, infused with blood and vitality. As you clasp their hand, you can feel it cooling. The remnants of life are physically, awfully, ebbing away.

Comprehending the moment of transition from life to death is hard enough, but Joe's task is of a different order of magnitude— and would have been unfathomable to Owen, who was killed in action in 1918, just one week before the Armistice brought an end to hostilities. Thanks to the medical advances of the twentieth century—in particular, to the invention of mechanical ventilation and intensive care in the 1950s—Keira is, or appears to be, simultaneously alive and dead. Her doctors are proposing one thing, yet

Joe's senses speak of something else entirely. She is literally breathing—her heart is literally beating. If he strokes her hand, her fingers clasp his, a reflex action that appears to be intentional. He is being asked to accept that his daughter may have no perceptible brain function, yet is able to move, metabolize, digest food, excrete waste, and persist for days, weeks, months, or years in a no-man's-land of mechanical life support, looking for all the world as though she is merely sleeping. It is too much, too hard to grasp.

The truth is, when the Danish anesthesiologist Bjørn Ibsen first began to mechanically ventilate children with polio in 1952, he unwittingly set in motion a chain of events no less revolutionary than those triggered by the great astronomer Nicolaus Copernicus, who in the sixteenth century overturned centuries of thought by positioning the sun, not the Earth, at the center of the universe. Copernican heliocentrism wasn't just radical; it was deeply uncomfortable and heretically contentious, defying centuries of Catholic doctrine that insisted the heavens revolved around the Earth. This relegation of God's creation was an assault on the authority of the Church itself; and as such, provoked a fearsome reaction. For the crime of championing Copernicus, for example, Galileo Galilei was tried by the Roman Inquisition in 1633, found "vehemently suspect of heresy," and forced to recant his views. He spent the rest of his life under house arrest.[8] Throughout the 1950s, in fledgling ICUs across the world, something equally epochal was beginning to unfold: the redefinition of death itself.

All Ibsen had cared about in 1952 was trying to prevent polio from claiming children's lives. He pushed air, by force, into paralyzed lungs simply to supply the oxygen without which, he knew, his young patients would die. But as with so many other medical innovations—from test-tube babies to genetic engineering, deep brain stimulation to retinal implants—the new technologies of intensive care began to raise profound questions about what it means to be alive, leaving bioethicists, lawyers, and governments racing to keep up. It took the audacity of two French professors of medicine—the neurologist Pierre Mollaret and the infectious diseases specialist Maurice Goulon—to propose in public for the first time that the era of death as a simple and unambiguous fact was over.[9]

In 1959, scientific breakthroughs came fast and furiously. A newly formed space agency, NASA, sent two monkeys into space and managed to bring them safely down to Earth again. The term "laser" was coined, the first bone marrow transplant performed, and a Russian spacecraft managed to photograph the far side of the moon. But the most groundbreaking moment of all occurred not in a fanfare of headlines, but quietly, discreetly, before an audience of medical men in dark flannel suits. The occasion was the twenty-second annual International Neurological Congress in Paris. When Mollaret and Goulon took to a podium before their academic peers, they knew full well that what they said next would rattle the foundations of medicine.[10] Perhaps the occasion—the sight of so many physicians of global renown—caused the pair to shuffle their papers and clear their throats in unease. Or perhaps the thought of the gauntlet they were about to throw down was a moment to savor and cherish.

In the terse and dispassionate terminology beloved of doctors, they began to describe the neurological features of a series of ventilated patients with catastrophic brain injuries in their ICU. Later, they would publish a paper in the *Revue Neurologique* describing twenty-three of the cases in more detail.[11] The patients had no discernible brain activity of any kind. In contrast to the rippling waveforms of a normal electroencephalogram (EEG) generated by electrical current in a healthy brain, their EEGs were flat, featureless. Crucially, even the part of the brain that connects our cerebral hemispheres to the spinal cord—the brain stem—was inert. This mattered because the brain stem contains the nerve tracts responsible for the movement and sensation of the entire body below the face, as well as the cranial nerves responsible for taste, smell, vision, and facial sensation. The brain stem is responsible for attention, the sleep-wake cycle, and consciousness. It even controls breathing. Human life is not possible, in short, without a functioning brain stem.

The patients described by Mollaret and Goulon had been subjected to rigorous clinical tests aimed at eliciting the most primal reflexes a human being possesses. To a painful stimulus: nothing. To the brush of cotton against the gossamer film that coats the eyeball: not so much as an eyelid's flicker. To disconnection from the ventilator and the near-lethal accumulation of carbon dioxide in the bloodstream: not the faintest effort to breathe unaided. These patients were not merely comatose, they had crossed into a penumbral state far beyond coma: one defined by the pair as *coma dépassé*, or "irreversible coma"—a term that would soon become synonymous with brain death.[12]

Mollaret and Goulon did not stop there. They took their observations all the way to their logical conclusions by pointing out that it was not just *unlikely* that these patients would ever be able to breathe without a ventilator, it was absolutely certain they would not. The necessary connections in the brain stem had completely ceased to function. Nor could they ever spontaneously recover consciousness—indeed, in some cases, the tissue of the brain stem and cerebral hemispheres was already decaying and liquefying. Without a ventilator, in short, these patients would already be dead. Yet for as long as they remained mechanically wedded to their Engström 150s, their hearts could continue to receive oxygen and beat indefatigably.

This posed a profound question. How could the continued ventilation of these patients be in their best interests? Without any prospect of recovery, further ventilation was surely futile?[13] In her book *The Ethics of Transplants*, the philosopher Janet Radcliffe Richards is characteristically blunt on this issue: "What, then, was the status of these patients? Were they being kept alive by the ventilator ('life support machine') or was the machine pumping oxygenated blood round a corpse?"[14]

Mollaret and Goulon were bold enough to supply an answer. Despite their beating hearts and pulsing blood, patients in a *coma dépassé* were already dead, they said—they could no longer be regarded as living. In their view, the heartbeat—for so many centuries the cardinal sign of vivacity—no longer defined the essence of life. Now a functioning brain was required. Just as Copernicus had located the sun, not the Earth, at the center of existence, so, too, had Mollaret and Goulon dethroned the heart and anointed the brain in its place. Modern death was a matter of neurology, not cardiology. The cessation of *brain* function was what counted.

It is hard to overstate how momentous these ideas must have seemed at the time. Until this point, when it came to matters of life and death, the heart had ruled supreme. Nor was the heart's pivotal role in our self-understanding an accident, with its exertions and responses to our fluctuating emotions being, literally, heartfelt. As the American cardiologist and author Sandeep Jauhar beautifully puts it in *Heart: A History*, his 2018 love letter to cardiology:

> Perhaps we associate the heart with life because, like life itself, the heart is dynamic. From second to second, and on a macroscopic level, the heart is the only organ that discernibly moves. Through its murmurings, it speaks to us; through its synchronized contractions, it broadcasts an electrical signal several thousand times more powerful than any other in the body.

The notion that the heart—so closely associated with courage, compassion, love, and desire, and for so long regarded as the seat of the soul—could continue to beat within the chest of a corpse was beyond controversial; it was almost profane. Yet this was because throughout human history, the crucial elements of life—heart, lungs, and brain—had always functioned or failed roughly simultaneously. With a handful of exceptions, the moment any one of this triad was fatally injured—through a bullet to the chest, a prolonged immersion in water, or a grievous head injury, for example—the other two swiftly followed suit. Mechanical ventilation had disrupted dying by preventing patients with calamitous head injuries from immediately tipping into respiratory and cardiac death—but only for as long as they remained hooked to a machine. Turn off the ventilator, and death was swift and absolute. In refusing to gloss over or flinch from the enormity of this transformation, Mollaret and Goulon were medical trailblazers. Their ideas were dizzying, electrifying—and they were going to revolutionize transplant surgery.

———

An amiable din fills the Bristol Royal Hospital for Children's pediatric intensive care unit. Children and adults—a rackety pack of them—have rushed from Devon to be at Keira's side. Her sisters, her grandparents, and her aunties are here, garrulous, restive, hoping for miracles. Neither Loanna nor Bradley are able to join them. Both are still recovering from their major surgeries. Joe, who until now has managed to keep command of his emotions, takes one look at Keely, his oldest child, and finds he is crying before he can speak. *It's quite bad* is all he can manage to utter. Keely, who has never seen her father cry before, stares at him as the words land, as fear begins to grip her heart and empty her lungs of air.

Both girls are desperate to see Keira. They rush into her room, effusive, and clamber into bed with their little sister. *Bob!* exclaims Katelyn. *Bob! We're here!* The nickname stands for Bobalobadingdong and no one in the family can quite remember its origin, except that somehow it is linked to Keira's passion for singing. The girls cover her shoulders with a fluffy white cardigan, tuck her favorite cuddly dog under her arm, and prop a phone against her pillow. With "Symphony" by Clean Bandit blasting out on repeat, they chatter unstoppably about hair, nails, horses, music, exactly as though it is a conversation all three of them are sharing. They soften Keira's lips with strawberry lip balm and gently elevate her hands in turn, painting each nail a dazzling shade of orange. Finally, with the easy skill that comes with much practice, they adorn her fingers with Haribo gummy rings—more highly prized than diamonds when you are nine years old.

What strikes Jemma Evans more than anything is how open with each other the Balls are. "They communicated completely honestly. That's quite unusual. They were dealing with it all together, not trying to shield the other children in the family from it. A lot of other parents in this kind of situation would try to keep the siblings away. Keira's family stands out because they absolutely didn't do that. And that was obviously how Joe and Loanna parented their children in normal times, with that openness and honesty. This was their normal family dynamic, which they kind of were able to continue in a time of great stress. The children weren't shielded, they weren't separated, they were there for everything."

Parents' instincts to try to protect their children from distress by providing little or no information about their hospitalized sibling are both well documented and shared by some healthcare professionals.[15] According to one study:

> Nurses may overlook siblings and assume parents and other family
> members are supporting them; however, distraught parents may
> not have the insight to identify the needs of their well children,
> not know how to explain the situation, or be unaware that well

siblings benefit from being with their ill sister or brother. Siblings frequently remain invisible, are relegated to the waiting room, are rushed in and out, or are sent home with relatives.[16]

Jemma, who has over twelve years' experience of pediatric critical-care nursing, believes that excluding siblings from the PICU, despite being well-meaning, can sometimes have adverse consequences. "I think children have incredible imaginations and what they imagine is often worse than reality. And so actually, including them and being honest with them means they're not imagining something even more painful." The evidence, though scant, seems to corroborate this, with studies demonstrating that when a child is in intensive care, an information void can sometimes accentuate the stress experienced by siblings.[17]

As Keely and Katelyn lavish care and attention on their unconscious sister, it would be easy to assume from their laughter, exuberance, and ceaseless chatter that they are simply too young to understand the gravity of her injuries. But that would be to do them a disservice. For their efforts, almost frenzied, to treat Keira as a living, loving, conscious sister stem not from naivete but from its opposite. Their eyes dart and rove as they monitor the nurses' every word and gesture. They listen, grasp, and absorb it all, the bleak and unforgiving facts of the matter. "Even though there were ten of us in Keira's room at one stage, I kept looking all the time at Keira," says Keely. "I kept hoping I'd notice something the doctors had missed, some little thing that showed she wasn't brain dead and I could tell them."

Katelyn is equally circumspect. If anyone was paying attention, they would have spotted her fingers, laid firmly and unwaveringly upon her sister's chest. Earlier, Katelyn overheard a nurse telling Joe that Keira's heart could stop beating at any time. Ever since, she has kept her hand in position, attuned to the cadence of Keira's ribs against her palm, poised to sound the alarm should that rhythm falter. It is an act of consuming vigilance. "But if I didn't do it, I thought her heart might stop and no one would realize," says Katelyn, who, far from being ignorant of her sister's fragility, is doing all she can to keep her alive. Never underestimate the clarity and intelligence of a child in a hospital. Throughout that Monday, Keely and Katelyn cuddle and talk to and pamper their sister not out of innocence, but precisely because it is intolerable to imagine the world without her in it.

As day wears into evening, Dr. Sarah Goodwin, the consultant responsible for the unit that night, begins her shift. An athletic mother of two, she is intense and sinewy, a coiled spring of energy. You sense she could stride through twenty-four-hour shifts on caffeine and willpower alone. Prior to entering Keira's room, Sarah has committed to memory the smallest details of her physiological state. Nothing about brain stem testing or the concept of brain death—let alone the idea of organ donation—has yet been broached with Joe. Today has been about giving a grieving family the space and time they need to focus on Keira and endeavor to comprehend the magnitude of her injuries. "I certainly wasn't planning on having an organ donation conversation that evening, not least because Loanna wasn't able to be there. I was really just going in to say hi and explain anything they didn't understand," Sarah recalls.

ICU doctors have a well-deserved reputation for being imperturbable in even the most harrowing of circumstances, but what happens next floors Sarah. In response to being asked if anyone in the family has any questions, Katelyn, who looks almost identical to Keira, turns her clear blue eyes on the doctor. "She looked directly at me and said, 'Can we donate her organs?'" says Sarah. "I looked straight back at her, because I was not expecting that at all, and then I said, 'Yes, absolutely. We will start looking into that for you, if that's what you would like us to do.' Then Katelyn turned to

Joe and said, 'Dad, we've got to do this because it's what she would have wanted. I know it's what she would have wanted.'"

It is Katelyn's maturity and eloquence that Sarah finds so arresting. Joe is still overwhelmed, clearly struggling to process the ordeal of the preceding twenty-four hours, yet Katelyn, despite being only eleven years old, is resolute. "She was so determined, she was just going to make this happen. She pushed it so clearly and calmly, she just led the whole thing, which is something I've never seen before—a child driving organ donation—but she was absolutely going to pull everyone along with her at that point. I had the sense that Joe couldn't even start to think about it for a moment, but that it didn't really matter because Katelyn was on a mission. Then Joe thought about it; he managed to get his head around it, too, and he said, 'Yes, yes she would. Of course she'd want to be an organ donor. Keira is the kind of girl who gives her last sweet to her sisters.'"

The force of Katelyn's desire to help her sister help others through donating her organs shatters the careful choreography with which the subject is normally navigated. In the UK, for example, clinical guidance for the identification of potential organ donors is codified by the National Institute for Health and Care Excellence (NICE).[18] The NICE guidance, updated in 2016 and based on the best available international evidence, is unequivocal in its direction of clinical teams. It advises that when a patient meets a specific set of criteria—namely, that they have had a catastrophic brain injury; that their GCS is 4 or lower and that this is not explained by sedation; that one or more cranial nerve reflexes is absent—then the patient should usually be considered as potentially suitable for organ donation. At this point, the guidance states: "The healthcare team caring for the patient should initiate discussions about potential organ donation with the specialist nurse in organ donation at the time the criteria are met."

Specialist nurses for organ donation, colloquially known as SNODs, are the bedrock of the UK's organ donation system. In the US, they are known more simply as transplant nurses. These highly skilled individuals receive exhaustive training in communication and family support, especially in conversations exploring a person's preferences around the end of life. Involving the SNOD early—right from the initial end-of-life care discussions—allows a relationship and rapport to develop between family and nurse, enabling the nurse to better support the family through the end-of-life care process. SNODs typically remain closely involved with a family all the way through to the retrieval of organs and beyond. They may help support a family through their bereavement process for months after their loved one has died. In addition to this vital, intensive family support, SNODs mastermind the intricate logistics necessary to ensure the successful transit and transplantation of organs from one body into another. They are required to be operational ninjas and superlative communicators. The role is both fiendishly challenging and exceptionally rewarding.

In Keira's case, the specialist nurse who will become critically important to the Ball family—and who will develop an enduring relationship with Joe, Loanna, Keely, Katelyn, and Bradley—is thirty-two-year-old Sarah Crosby. Sarah has the kind of friendly, open, guileless face that makes you feel you can share your innermost feelings after all of two minutes of chatting. With blond hair and frank eyes, she exudes warmth and understanding. Even as a newly minted nurse, in her very first placement in an eye clinic, Sarah was intoxicated by the possibilities of transplant nursing. "I was one of the nurses trained to do corneal retrieval from people who had died and wished to be donors," she recalls. "The fact that we could restore somebody's sight by retrieving a person's eyes was absolutely fascinating to me. I deliberately took steps to gain experience in the emergency department and ICU because I just knew I wanted to become a specialist for organ donation. I changed my career to make that happen."

Some people recoil from the idea of discussing organ donation with a family still reeling from the worst news imaginable, but Sarah sees these conversations less as daunting than as a positive opportunity to help families. "In the back of my mind, I know nothing I say can make their day any worse because they've already lost their loved one. This is the worst day of their life. But if I can give them a slight bit of hope and comfort by offering organ donation as a part of end-of-life care, then that's what I need to do. It's not a taboo topic. It's a normal part of critical care. If someone meets the criteria to be an organ donor and we're not offering it to them, then I'm not doing my patient justice, I'm not being their advocate. The foundation of who I am as a nurse is trying to support the family however I can. Organ donation can help a family feel as though something good has come out of an awful situation, so it can be incredibly positive."

The timing of the initial conversation is critical. If it occurs too soon, when a patient has only just arrived in hospital, the family's grief may be too intense for them to contemplate donation. If it occurs too late, when life-sustaining treatment is about to be withdrawn, then a twenty-four-hour period of intricate medical assessment and logistics—vital to determining whether someone is or is not suitable to be a donor—is lost. The ideal time is shortly after a family has understood and accepted that their loved one is going to die, and that there is no way of saving them. At that point, if appropriate, Sarah might raise organ donation alongside other aspects of end-of-life care—the making of handprints, the preserving of locks of hair, and whether the family would like chaplaincy involved, for example. Typically, the starting point is not donation itself, but the personality and wishes of the patient. What kind of person are they? What matters to them most? Did they ever express a view on organ donation? "There's no big drama, it's just another optional part of end-of-life care to discuss. It's not for everybody, but it is my duty to raise it," says Sarah.

At 2:46 a.m. on Tuesday, August 1, Sarah Goodwin picks up the phone and calls the national Organ Donation and Transplant Hub, the nerve center through which every transplant is coordinated across the whole of the UK. She informs the coordinator on the other end of the line that there may be a prospective pediatric donor in Bristol. It is the briefest of conversations. *We are nowhere near testing*, Sarah explains, *but the family would like to speak to a SNOD in due course.* The coordinator carefully enters Keira's basic details into a database of potential donors and alerts the SNOD on call that night for Bristol—a colleague of Sarah Crosby's—to the need to meet Joe the next morning. These are early days, tiny steps—no more, really, than a slow and creaking tectonic rumble—but if momentum builds, if the stars align, then a vast team of geographically distant surgeons, physicians, perfusionists, pilots, coordinators, porters, anesthesiologists, and nurses may end up toiling, sweating, clamping, and dissecting until at last, against the clock, in multiple operating theaters around the country, the tragedy of Keira's death is sublimated, against the odds, into new life.

It is for this reason that Sarah Goodwin, just like Sarah Crosby, regards discussions about organ donation not as a burden, but as a privilege. "I believe that they are about giving the family in front of me solace. I go on to see these families down the line for bereavement follow-up. I can tell you that nobody I've spoken to has ever regretted saying yes to organ donation. It's the opposite, it gives families a huge amount of hope. It is the one good thing, the one extraordinary thing, that can come out of such terrible tragedies."

HeartWare

A few days after his ninth birthday, Max Johnson was blue-lit by ambulance to the Cardiothoracic Unit at Newcastle's Freeman Hospital. For all his gauntness and pallor, his entrance was by no means a quiet one. With his ever-expanding collection of loudspeakers blaring techno beats across his cubicle, the pediatric intensive care team settled Max into bed. Before long, the doctors and nurses were making him laugh with a loud and raucous impromptu dance party that possibly owed more to enthusiasm than to anyone's innate sense of rhythm. "From that moment on, Max was forever associated with his love of music and speakers," recalls his father, Paul. It was not that the team was unaware of how desperately sick and unstable Max was, but that the fear rolled off him in waves. They could see that what he needed, in addition to the infusions of inotropes and meticulous monitoring, was intensive care of the human spirit. The team was showing a frightened little boy that, in this moment, in this unit, ICU stood for "I see you"—that they were loving, and silly, and kind.

A cardiology registrar performed an echocardiogram to assess how effectively Max's heart was functioning. Stooped in silence over Max's chest, the doctor directed the probe across the contours of each of the four chambers in turn, while studying their two-dimensional re-creation on-screen. His verdict, though it came as no surprise, left

Paul reeling. "He said the heart function was terrible. It was a shock to hear. But, unfortunately, how else can it be done? We're all perhaps guilty of telling the odd white lie in response to a question, to spare feelings. This isn't something you can do when you are talking about the viability of someone's life. You can't offer false hope. The function of Max's heart was terrible. That was the reality."

Max was sufficiently stable overnight for the PICU team to transfer him downstairs in the morning to the Children's Heart Unit. The unit, otherwise known as Ward 23, cares for critically unwell children with heart and lung conditions from across the whole of the UK and Ireland, though the majority come from the north of England. With twenty beds, six of which are high-dependency beds acting as a halfway house between intensive care and ordinary ward care, the Children's Heart Unit is one of only two centers in the UK to carry out pediatric heart transplants. Depending on the severity of their illnesses, children can spend days, weeks, or months on the ward. Unbeknownst to Max, he was destined to become one of its longest-staying patients.

Later that afternoon, the clinical lead for the Freeman's pediatric heart transplant service, a consultant pediatric cardiologist named Dr. Zdenka Reinhardt, invited Max's parents to sit down and talk. "We made our way in silence to a room tucked around the corner at the end of the ward," says Paul. "Even in this first meeting, you could appreciate her fierce intellect. Although she spoke to us with honesty and frankness, her eyes were full of compassion and kindness. She understood that her words were hitting us with devastating force. After all, she had done this many, many times before." As Paul and Emma fidgeted nervously on turquoise plastic seats—Paul digging his fingers into his thigh to try to stop his leg jiggling—Zdenka began to put shape to Max's future.

First, for the next three to five days, he would be exhaustively assessed for suitability for transplant. Part of the assessment would be psychosocial: both the surgery and its aftermath would be punishing experiences that demanded mental as well as physical resilience. The results would be collated and discussed at the next multidisciplinary transplant assessment meeting, when the decision would be made whether or not to list Max for transplant. A place on the waiting list would by no means guarantee him a new heart. Unlike other organs, hearts and lungs must be matched by size in children because of limited space inside the chest cavity, and to ensure the two organs have comparable strength and do not overwhelm or underpower the other. This means that children wait two and a half times as long as adults for an urgent heart transplant.[1] In the UK, one in every eight children dies before an organ becomes available.[2]

If this were not daunting enough, the most unpalatable truth that Zdenka needed to convey was that a heart transplant, for all its extraordinary ability to save a child on the brink of death, was simultaneously an act of last resort—something that Max's doctors would avoid if they possibly could. This was not because donor organs were in desperately short supply (though they are), or because the surgery was a grueling and dangerous assault on the body (though it is), but because a heart transplant consigns a patient to a future of lifelong—and life-shortening—jeopardy. The average life expectancy of a patient after a heart transplant in the UK is fourteen years, though occasionally patients may live for double that period.[3] In the specific circumstances Max was likely to face—a first pediatric heart transplant from a donor after brain death—9 percent of children do not survive the first year and 18 percent do not survive the first five years.[4]

Paul and Emma listened in silence as Zdenka explained how the permanent immunosuppression required after a heart transplant increases the recipient's risk of cancer, renal failure, prematurely blocked coronary arteries, and—hanging over them all—the ever-present menace of the body rejecting its new heart. It was for this reason, she said, that a heart transplant should not really be thought of as a cure but as a palliative treatment. "Emma and I just looked at one another, and Emma burst into tears," says Paul. "We had just been presented with our new best-case scenario—our lives were changed forever. The grief we were feeling for our son and the lives we had known was like a weight dragging us to the bottom of a very deep, dark, cold place. Transplantation was the option when there is no option." Later, as Paul drove back home with Harry, he tried to convey to his eleven-year-old son what Zdenka had communicated. Immediately grasping all that Max had lost—the blithe promise of youth, the presumed sunny future—Harry wept in the back of the car.

On January 18, 2017, Max Johnson was placed on the UK's pediatric heart transplant list. The NHS is careful to stress that a transplant waiting list is not a queuing system in which the next person in line is offered the next available organ. Rather, it is a matching system in which multiple criteria such as the size, age, and health of the donor and the recipient, how closely their blood and tissue types match, and the urgency of need of the various patients on the list must all be finely balanced. To the parents and children whose lives are on hold, though, the list can often feel like the most pitiless queue in the world. Everyone has joined a club whose members are being whittled by deadly attrition. On the ward, you quickly come to know and care about the other children awaiting new hearts of their own, the other parents whose lives are also in free fall. Time passes. The first of the other children dies. More time, then another, and then another. All the while you hope and pray and beg and bargain that somehow—you would give your own life to make it happen—a heart for your child will arrive in time. One day a phrase leapt out at Paul: "A look at the notes at the end of Max's bed spelled it out in simple, honest language. Max had 'end-stage heart failure.' End-stage. We were at the buffers with nowhere else to go."

———

Members of staff have a secret weapon in a children's hospital, and that weapon is play. When Max arrived at the Freeman in 2017, Joanne Moore had over eighteen years' experience as a Ward 23 play specialist. She saw immediately how anxious and overwhelmed Max was as he mutely observed the ward around him. "He was very quiet. You could see he didn't know what was going on. But we are really good at adapting to individual children's needs, and once we knew how much he loved music, we helped him set up his speakers in a corner of the playroom." Every so often, Joanne would take Max with his wheelchair and drip stand into the playroom so he could enjoy a blast of loud music and disco lights. "It's amazing how helpful it can be to spend time in the playroom. If you're just sitting on the floor chatting, a child feels more relaxed and might open up to you about what's worrying them. We're not like the nurses or the doctors. We don't do anything invasive like blood tests or cannulas. Our role is all about friendship building and relationship building."

As well as developing a strong rapport with children and their parents, and helping them feel safe enough to confide their fears, play specialists use play to explain to children what will happen to them, especially during medical procedures. With younger children, this could be via the use of dolls or books, but with Max it entailed answering a never-ending stream of questions. "Max was very intelligent and very inquisitive. I remember he needed a CT scan, so we went down beforehand to have a look at the machine and he asked so many questions, even the radiographer didn't know all the answers." You never know what will pique a child's curiosity, says Joanne. One young child, on discussing his imminent heart surgery, had only one burning question, which was what color thread he would be sewn up with afterward. Another little boy, around six years old, was waiting for a heart transplant when a friend from his school came to visit. The classmate was perplexed by one thing in particular. "He really loves fish fingers," he told Joanne. "But after he has his new heart, will he still like fish fingers?"

Emma and Paul were fortunate enough to be given accommodation in a building on the hospital site called Scott House, funded by a charity called the Sick Children's Trust. It meant that for the duration of Max's stay in hospital—which they still imagined would be a few weeks long—one or another of them could always be by his side without the family incurring stratospheric hotel bills. Nevertheless, the logistics of parenting one child in a hospital that was nearly two hundred miles away from where the other child went to school remained grueling. Emma and Paul adopted a tag-team approach, taking turns to spend half a week with Max in hospital, then the other half at home with Harry. The Wetherby Services rest stop on the A1 highway became a dismal twice-weekly rendezvous point where husband and wife would meet, snatch a coffee, briefly embrace, then disappear into opposite lanes of traffic, destined not to meet in person again for another three or four days.

"Being the parent of a very sick child can be a lonely, isolating experience," says Paul, whose nightmares were unrelenting. By 5 a.m. he would be wide-awake, his foot drumming compulsively against the mattress and his stomach knotted with dread. Nauseous hours would pass. Only when he had called Max and heard the sound of his voice would the fear slither away. Max, on the other hand, initially remained surprisingly cheerful, even managing on a good day to slick back his hair with gel and negotiate a shower with a waterproof speaker and a drip stand. "The thing that always amazes me is children's resilience," says Joanne. "We do these incredible things to them like put machines in their hearts, but they still want to play, still want to do their schoolwork, still have this spirit that comes from nowhere. I think if it was us, we'd probably be lying in bed feeling very sorry for ourselves, but children go for surgery and the next day they have this inbuilt attitude of 'Oh, we like to play, we like to be busy, we like to be doing things, and if we can, we will.'"

A devoted team of nurses, doctors, play specialists, teachers, psychologists, physiotherapists, healthcare assistants, and the ward cleaner, Barbara, rallied around Max, trying to keep his spirits buoyant. The ward even had regular visits from clown doctors—local actors whose skits in white coats and red noses made Max laugh out loud despite himself. But he was never well enough to leave one of the ward's six high-dependency beds, and his weight continued to drop. He took to spending long periods staring out the window at a beech tree surrounded by grass, which he christened the "Tree of Life." One day, a nurse noticed him crying as he stared at the tree. She asked what was wrong and he replied simply, "I hope that I'll be able to go outside again one day." By the end of January, despite every effort to coax him to eat, Max was so emaciated that he was at risk of being too frail to remain on the transplant list. He required feeding via a nasogastric tube, the insertion of which was so traumatic that afterward he spent several days sitting motionless, staring out the window. "It felt to Emma as if he had lost a piece of his soul," says Paul. "His eyes were glazed over and his spark was snuffed out. The crushing realization that someone you love so unconditionally is suffering and you can't stop it is terrible."

On the evening of February 1, one of the consultant cardiothoracic surgeons looking after Max, Fabrizio De Rita, came to review him. The unexpected visit—he had been once already on his morning ward round—immediately worried Emma, who was there at the bedside. A new consultant, two years into the role, Fabrizio had studied medicine in his home country of Italy, then moved to the UK for his specialist training. A young, enthusiastic surgeon with close-cropped hair, dense stubble, and a wide, easy smile, he had been carefully monitoring Max's trajectory ever since his first day at the Freeman. "For adult patients, the decline is well-defined. We know what we need to watch, where the limits are, when we need to consider artificial support like putting a pump in. But in kids, it's way more challenging. They can't always tell you how unwell they feel. You have to watch them and recognize the signs and symptoms that might potentially trigger a very rapid deterioration. They don't breathe as easily, they don't eat as much. Long before becoming unwell, they lose energy. They're not able to perform as before. It can be very difficult to tease these things out, and the problem with children is they tend to keep on being able to cope, but then suddenly they crash very quickly."

In the absence of a donor organ—and with no idea when one might materialize—the dilemma faced by Fabrizio and his team was whether to implant a mechanical pump into Max's heart in order to assist artificially with the job of driving the circulation. Without such a pump, called a ventricular assist device, they knew Max was at risk of multi-organ failure. When the left ventricle—the largest and most powerful of the heart's four chambers—is unable to contract forcefully, as in Max's case, it cannot expel blood at speed into the aorta. The patient's blood pressure consequently plummets until any part of the body whose functioning is particularly dependent on abundant supplies of oxygen, such as the kidneys, begins to fail. Worse, the blood that the heart is too weak to expel begins to back up inside the veins, causing harmful congestion in the lungs and liver. This means that four separate organ systems are under pressure at once—heart, lungs, liver, and kidneys—a perilous state for the patient. "Max was already receiving the maximum dose of milrinone to support the circulation, but the blood tests we'd done suggested worsening functioning of the other organs like his kidneys and liver," says Fabrizio. "His echocardiogram was shocking. It was showing us the left side of his heart was extremely dilated and not really moving at all. In these circumstances, you can predict that something's going to happen. He was on the razor's edge. He was going to collapse and suffer a cardiac arrest."

Even with the very real threat of a cardiac arrest, the decision whether to implant a VAD was by no means straightforward. Foreign bodies in the heart, such as a mechanical pump or a metal replacement valve, drastically increase the likelihood of blood clots and hence the risk to the patient of suffering a stroke. The Berlin Heart, for example—the only kind of VAD that is specifically manufactured for children—has such a high stroke risk that around one in three children who are connected to the device for a year will experience a stroke.[5] If they are lucky, the strokes will be mild; if unlucky, they may cause permanent disability or death. To try to reduce the risk, patients with VADs are placed on medications that make it harder for the blood to clot, but anticoagulants introduce a new risk—one of unwanted, sometimes life-threatening, bleeding. Max was fortunate in that he was just big enough to be able to avoid a Berlin Heart and have, instead, an adult VAD known as a HeartWare device, which would lower his stroke risk. Nevertheless, he would still face a one-in-six chance of a stroke for every year that the device was implanted.[6]

That evening, when Fabrizio laid his stethoscope on Max's chest, his heart was so grossly distended—and laboring so furiously to beat—that the drum of the stethoscope physically bounced up and down on his ribs. Max was hot, panting, gasping for air, too breathless now even to speak. Away from his bedside, Fabrizio sat down with Emma to explain why he felt they had no choice but to act immediately. "Fabrizio could see that Max's heart was literally pounding out of his chest," says Emma. "He said, 'We can't wait any longer. We need to do this in the morning because Max is really struggling.' Nobody actually said he could die at any moment, but he produced the consent papers and went through it there and then."

The VAD was intended to be a "bridge to transplant"—a means of keeping Max alive on the transplant waiting list for as long as it took to find a match. In truth, it was a necessary evil, a device that could potentially harm him, but without which he was likely to die. These were the odds that surgeons like Fabrizio weighed daily—the mortal costs of inaction versus action. An impossible conundrum, algebra with no known solution, in which x always stands for uncertainty. They could draw on all their years of expertise, the children saved, the children lost, but in the end—and what a burden to live with—it could only come down to a well-informed gamble. "These procedures are only ever done when children are critically ill. We have to try and explain that we hope it will be successful, but their child's journey might end at any stage because of potential complications," says Fabrizio. "We explain numbers and statistics based on the evidence and our experiences—but of course for the parents it is always zero or a hundred percent, because how can they accept the percentages? It is the life of one single person that matters."

As Emma tried to comprehend all she was being told, one thing gave her solace. "Fabrizio was gentle. That gentle nature was important. He was very humble. Whenever I spoke to him, I could tell he genuinely cared about Max, and that made me hopeful." Humility—not a quality typically associated with cardiothoracic surgeons—made Emma feel that she could trust Fabrizio, and that Max was safe in his hands.

The next morning, the hospital's VAD coordinator came to show Max and his parents what a HeartWare device looked like. The size and shape of a mushroom, the £90,000 titanium pump would be surgically stitched into the wall of Max's failing left ventricle, from where it would divert blood away from the heart through a small plastic tube, then back into the aorta. Inside the pump, a solid gold impeller—or frictionless motor—would propel the blood by spinning at three thousand revolutions per minute, generating up to ten liters per minute of blood flow. The exquisite engineering of a beating heart has yet to be matched by anything built by human hands, but the HeartWare device perhaps came close. Once successfully sealed within the cave of Max's chest, the pump would be connected to an external controller and two lithium battery packs, via a wire exiting the body through the upper abdomen. When he woke up, he would be a boy without a pulse. Continuously flowing, mechanically driven blood would course instead through his body.

Max turned the shiny object over and over in his hands, marveling at its smoothness and the glint of gold within. Titanium, lithium, gold—it all seemed so high-tech as to be almost exciting. "I think it was a novelty for Max, this special metal thing that would go inside his chest to help him. We saw it as a positive, too, something he needed that the doctors could do for him," says Emma. "I don't think I even realized that this was going to be open-heart surgery or what that meant, how big and serious an operation this was going to be. It hadn't registered that they were going to cut open his sternum. I had no idea about the bypass machine, either. It just went over my head." Paul, like Emma, was largely oblivious. "We really had no idea about the enormity of the surgery. I remember staring in wonder at this little thing sitting on Max's bedside locker, thinking, 'Wow, this is going to pump blood around his body.' I knew he'd be on a machine during the surgery to oxygenate his blood, so I understood the mechanics, but what I didn't understand in any shape or form was the scale of that. When we first saw Max after he came back from theater, it utterly took the wind out of our sails. It floored us."

It was a blessing, perhaps, that despite Fabrizio's sensitive and compassionate explanations, neither Emma nor Paul truly grasped what Max's surgery was going to entail, let alone the tortuous history that had led to this point, of valiant efforts, outlandish innovations, ferocious obsessions, and maverick surgeries that all too often, in the early days of cardiac surgery, cost patients their lives. The notion of using an external machine to perform the vital work of the heart and lungs, for example, was inconceivable at the start of the twentieth century. Then, surgeons could not even fathom how to stitch back together the severed ends of a blood vessel without the blood oozing out from within, let alone contemplate building an artificial pumping device.

———

In between divorcing and beheading assorted wives in the sixteenth century, Henry VIII is recorded as having once proclaimed that "no carpenter, smith, weaver or woman shall practise surgery."[7] When, in 1540, he granted the royal charter that founded the Company of Barber-Surgeons in the city of London, women were duly barred.[8] Their natural manual dexterity may have made them good at sewing, but not, heaven forbid, surgery. By the mid-nineteenth century, the behavior of upstart agitators like Elizabeth Garrett Anderson— destined, in 1865, to become the first woman in Britain to qualify as a doctor—led the *British Medical Journal* to issue a thundering editorial on the vexed matter of "the female doctor question":

> It is high time that this unnatural and preposterous attempt
> on the part of one or two highly strong-minded women to
> establish a race of feminine doctors should be exploded. How
> is it possible, in accordance with any of the notions of propriety
> and of sentiment which we feel towards the female sex in this
> country, for any man of proper feeling to sit by the side of a lady
> at a dissecting-table or in an anatomical lecture-room?[9]

Today, though women make up over 50 percent of medical students in the UK and the US, less than 10 percent of cardiothoracic surgeons in each country are female.[10] In such a male-dominated profession, it is perhaps ironic that one of the crucial figures in the history of heart transplantation is a female French embroiderer from the nineteenth century named Marie-Anne Leroudier. One of the finest embroiderers of her day, Leroudier was astonished when, in 1901, a young surgical trainee named Alexis Carrel came knocking on her door in Lyon, the home of the French silk industry. Like the rest of his fellow countrymen and -women, Carrel had been horrified when, in 1894, the French president Marie François Sadi Carnot was assassinated while visiting Lyon.[11] The assassin, an Italian anarchist, had deployed as his murder weapon a dagger disguised in a rolled-up newspaper. Darting out of the crowds that had congregated to glimpse the president, he stabbed him in the back, lacerating the portal vein. At the time, the only technique available to surgeons to staunch the flow from severed blood vessels was that of tying off, or ligating, the vessel. But the portal vein brought blood from the stomach and intestines to the liver—it was crucial to the functioning of life. Unable to ligate the vessel, the president's surgeons looked on helplessly as he bled to death before them.[12]

The president's assassination unleashed a storm of violence against Italian businesses, cafés, and homes across Lyon. But the object of Carrel's ire was closer to home: the impotence of his profession.[13] Had his surgical colleagues possessed the wherewithal to repair damaged blood vessels, the president might still be alive. But medical consensus held that creating a vascular anastomosis—surgically connecting two blood vessels using needle and thread—was impossible. Carrel was determined to change this, believing that if he could hone and refine current suturing practice, he would find a way to reunite the ends of severed blood vessels. With access to a laboratory at his hos-

pital in Lyon containing live dogs and surgical equipment—the ethics of animal vivisection at this time were opaque and largely left up
to self-regulation by medics[14]—Carrel swiftly discovered that suturing together two slippery, spaghetti-like vessels was going to require
novel techniques and equipment. The needles and threads used by
surgeons at the time were simply too bulky and crude for tiny blood
vessels, tending to tear them and risk the formation of blood clots.[15]

For the more sophisticated approach required, Carrel turned to
Lyon's famous embroidery district. In a local haberdashery whole-
saler he found delicate "No. 13 Kirby" needles from Birmingham,
UK, and gossamer-fine "Coton d'Alsace, No. 500" thread. Coating
both needle and thread in Vaseline helped them glide less traumat-
ically through vessels. But it was embroidery lessons from Marie-
Anne Leroudier that gave Carrel the manual dexterity to master
a technique of seamlessly suturing vessel to vessel, as described in
Spare Parts, historian Paul Craddock's history of transplantation:
"Through his lessons with Leroudier, he got to know what it felt like
to puncture a vessel in just the right way, to know when it was about
to tear, buckle, or give way. He knew just how far he could push his
materials and how the fabric of the human body would respond to
the action of his nimble, sensitive fingers."[16]

In 1902, Carrel disseminated his groundbreaking techniques
for creating vascular anastomoses in print and at scientific confer-
ences.[17] Tantalizingly, he also revealed that he was already using
the new techniques to experiment with transplanting the thyroid,
kidney, and pancreas from one dog into another. Shortly afterward, Carrel moved to the Rockefeller Institute in Chicago, where
he began working with an American surgeon, Charles Guthrie, to
further advance the possibilities of transplantation in animals. The
pair's macabre dog surgeries included swapping the legs of a black
dog with those of a white dog, and even, on one occasion, removing

the heart of one dog and sewing it into the neck of another, where it continued to beat for two hours.[18] In 1912, at the age of thirty-nine, Carrel became the youngest-ever recipient of the Nobel Prize in medicine for his pioneering work in vascular suturing. More than any individual to date, he had laid the foundations for the transplantation of human organs to be a realistic goal.

For all the radical surgical possibilities opened up by Alexis Carrel, the barriers to advancing open-heart surgery in the early twentieth century remained as daunting and seemingly insurmountable as ever. Even accessing the organ was an ordeal. Hidden beneath its citadel of bone and sinew, the only way to reach the whole of the heart was to saw through the sternum from top to bottom, then use a metal rib retractor to open a cavity. Wrenching the ribs apart using a hand-cranked pair of metal arms—a device scarcely changed since its invention in 1914[19]—was violent and destructive work. Of the 2 million people a year who have open-heart surgery today, for example, it is estimated that between 10 and 34 percent of patients end up with rib fractures.[20] Nerves can be crushed, ligaments ripped apart, and patients left with debilitating chronic pain. Worse, once the fortifications protecting the heart have been surgically breached, the lungs—no longer tethered to the inner thorax—invariably collapse, putting the patient at risk of respiratory failure.

The greatest challenge of all, though, for the earliest open-heart surgeons was how to operate with delicacy and finesse on an entity that insisted on leaping, contorting, bulging, and gyrating like a sack of rats fighting for freedom. Those surgeons' frantic grabs at bullets and shrapnel, timed between the contractions of a perpetually moving target, were both heroic and astonishingly effective, given the circumstances. But cardiac surgery was destined to be a dead-end craft unless its proponents could find a way to do the unthinkable: to stop the very organ whose motion was a prerequisite for life.

The human body is more robust than we tend to assume. In general, we have a surprising degree of built-in resilience to lack of food, water, and even oxygen. None of the cells from which we are built die instantaneously when their blood flow—and hence oxygen supply—is cut off. Even those parts of the body containing major muscle groups, such as the arms and legs, can successfully be reattached some six or eight hours after a traumatic amputation, for example, particularly if the severed limb is protected by being placed on ice.[21] The brain, however, unlike many other parts of the body, including the muscles, has no ability to store energy.[22] It is also highly metabolically active and thus exquisitely sensitive to oxygen. The intracranial circulation only has to be interrupted for two or three minutes before the onset of cellular injury. At normal temperatures, most of us are dead at six minutes.

The brain's voracious need for oxygen posed an intractable dilemma for pioneering cardiac surgeons. Their longing to engage more meticulously with the inner anatomy of the heart—potentially repairing complex wounds, congenital deformities, and valvular defects—required time. Yet for as long as the heart was opened up and the circulation interrupted, the patient risked hypoxic brain damage. What was needed was a means of prolonging the longevity of brain cells in the absence of oxygen, or of providing an artificial circulation to nourish the brain and other organs. There was an obvious candidate for the first approach. For centuries, hypothermia had been known to have therapeutic properties. Hippocrates noted that abandoned infants exposed to the open air survived longer in the cold winter months than in summer, and physicians in ancient Egypt, Rome, and Greece recommended inducing cooling for a wide variety of battlefield injuries and cerebral disturbances.[23] Cooling the body had the effect of lowering the metabolic activity of cells and tissues, significantly reducing their oxygen requirements.

The first surgeon to consider applying this principle to operating on an open heart was a Canadian named Wilfred Bigelow, whose inspiration cannot have been unrelated to his experiences amputating the gangrenous fingertips of patients who fell victim to the frostbitten depths of Canadian winter. On a research fellowship to Johns Hopkins Hospital in Baltimore to work with the pioneering American heart surgeon Alfred Blalock, Bigelow wrestled with how to give surgeons easier and longer access to the heart. "One night I awoke with a simple solution to the problem, and one that did not require pumps and tubes—cool the whole body, reduce the oxygen requirements, interrupt the circulation and open the heart."[24] After three years of testing his cooling theory on dogs in a laboratory, he used it successfully on a patient for the first time in 1952. Later, in a 1973 interview, Bigelow recalled the experience: "I remember the first time we cooled a patient. I think there must have been 28 people in the operating room and there was a great big fan blowing air over two large blocks of ice to keep the operating room cool. And it was great! Great excitement!"[25] Such surgeries were nail-biting affairs in which the anesthetized patient was first submerged in a cool bath into which ice cubes were poured until their body temperature had fallen to around 82.4 degrees Fahrenheit. Having been thoroughly dried, the patient's chest would be opened and clamps applied to the heart's major blood vessels, giving the surgeon a bloodless window of around eight to ten minutes in which to operate before the patient risked irreversible brain damage.

Hypothermia gave heart surgeons valuable additional operating time and is still used today as an adjunct to open-heart surgery. But a more definitive resolution of the problem was needed, and that lay in designing an artificial circulation to temporarily take over the work of the heart and lungs in theater. The doctor who would devote a quarter of a century to achieving precisely this was inspired to do so by one hellish night of medical impotence during which he could only look on from the bedside as a patient's life ebbed away.

John Gibbon was a junior surgical trainee when, in 1931, a fifty-three-year-old woman developed a life-threatening blood clot, a pulmonary embolism, after routine surgery.[26] The clot had blocked her pulmonary arteries, meaning that blood pumped from the heart struggled to enter the lungs. A senior surgeon moved the patient into an operating theater so that if her heart stopped, a large team on standby could attempt drastic emergency surgery to evacuate the clot. Gibbon remained at her side to monitor her condition for the next seventeen hours.[27] During this haunting vigil, he watched her deteriorate until, early the next morning, her heart, as predicted, ceased to beat. The surgical team sprang into action, but she died on the table shortly afterward. Years later, Gibbon still vividly recalled the experience:

> During that long night, helplessly watching the patient struggle for her life as her blood became darker and her veins more distended, the idea naturally occurred to me that if it were possible to remove continuously some of the blue blood from the patient's swollen veins, put oxygen into that blood and allow carbon dioxide to escape from it, and then to inject continuously the now-red blood back into the patient's arteries, we might have saved her life.[28]

Although he initially hoped to use such a device to save the lives of patients with massive pulmonary emboli, Gibbon had unwittingly just described the modern heart-lung machines, whose use today, in tens of thousands of operating theaters across the world, enables open-heart surgery. It would take him twenty-three years of laborious and obsessive work to get there. While not the first person to attempt to build a cardiopulmonary bypass machine, Gibbon was certainly the most dogged. He engineered pump after pump throughout the 1930s and '40s, learning, in the words of one cardio-thoracic surgeon, "to decipher every aspect of artificial circulation we now take for granted: how to drain the blood from the body, how to pump it back, how to clear air from the inside of the heart, how to anticoagulate successfully without clotting the machinery."[29] Particular challenges included the fragility of red blood cells, which are prone to bursting unless handled delicately, and the fact that when blood leaves the body and comes into contact with air, it clots.

Even if a pump could be devised that was sufficiently powerful to propel blood into every crevice of the human body without destroying red blood cells, replicating the function of the lungs outside the body was another monumental task. The lungs' cardinal role is that of gas exchange: they enable the removal of carbon dioxide from the blood, while replenishing red cells with fresh supplies of oxygen. In order to do so, during each inhalation we draw air down the large airways—the trachea and the two main bronchi—and into increasingly tiny bronchioles, each of which ends in a series of miniature air sacs known as alveoli. Clustered together like grapes on a vine, the alveoli are exceptionally thin-walled and surrounded by fine blood capillaries. As blood flows past, the wafer-thin barrier between blood and air permits the diffusion of carbon dioxide out of red cells and into the alveoli, and of oxygen into the blood from the opposite direction. What is remarkable about the whole process is how vast a surface area it involves. One typical human lung contains 240 million alveoli.[30] Collectively, they provide an internal surface area for gas exchange of around 430 square feet.[31] If a pair of lungs was unraveled so that the membranes of every alveolus were laid flat, they would cover an entire soccer field. Gibbon faced the small matter of designing an artificial equivalent.

With characteristic resolve, he chose to experiment initially on the stray cats that overran his home city of Philadelphia, since his prototype machine was too small to use on larger animals. He was forced to undertake forays into the suburbs under the cover of darkness to keep his laboratory well stocked with subjects: "Armed with a piece of tuna and a sack, Gibbon took to the streets at night, returning to the laboratory each time with a fresh supply of feral cats."[32] On May 6, 1953, twenty-two years after first embarking on the project, the indefatigable Gibbon finally performed the world's first successful open-heart operation using cardiopulmonary bypass. For twenty-six minutes, a critically ill eighteen-year-old college student named Cecelia Bavolek was kept alive on a heart-lung machine the size of a piano while Gibbon repaired a large atrial septal defect, or hole in her heart. She made a perfect recovery.[33] Gibbon's next two patients, each of them five years old, were less fortunate. Neither survived their operation, and after their deaths Gibbon chose never to operate on another human heart again. Nevertheless, his astonishing achievement in designing and building the first working heart-lung machine is regarded by many cardiac surgeons today as the single greatest milestone in the history of their craft.[34]

Over the next two years, various teams sought to build on Gibbon's work, the most successful of which was led by Clarence Walton Lillehei, a formidable cardiac surgeon at the University of Minnesota whose can-do attitude to the challenges and impediments holding back his specialty was exemplified by his comment "What mankind can dream, research and technology can achieve."[35] By 1954, Lillehei had already carried out forty-five open-heart surgeries in children using a technique known as "cross-circulation" to provide his young patients with oxygen. His inspiration was the role of the placenta in providing oxygenated blood from a mother's lungs to her developing baby in the womb. Similarly, Lillehei aimed to connect the circulations of a small creature (a young child needing open-heart surgery) to a larger one (most likely their parent) so that the parent could effectively breathe for both of them.[36]

After practicing exhaustively on dogs, Lillehei moved on to his first human subject. The patient was a one-year-old boy with a hole in his heart (a ventricular septal defect, in this case) named Gregory Glidden. His father, who shared Gregory's blood group, had volunteered to act as the donor.[37] Once both patients were anesthetized, large cannulas were used to feed Gregory's blood out of his body and into a vein in his father's leg. From there, father and child's blood intermingled as it was pumped up through the father's heart and lungs, receiving fresh oxygen, before being fed back into Gregory's aorta. No one in the operating theater was unaware that in this particular surgical procedure, the mortality rate could be 200 percent. For the next nineteen minutes, father breathed for son while Lillehei raced to cut into a heart that was little bigger than a strawberry, repair the hole within, and sew the heart back up again. One of the surgeons present later reflected in awe at what he had witnessed. "I am compelled to say that even now the opportunity to peer into the interior of a living beating human heart for the first time was one of the most momentous, moving, and humbling experiences I have ever had. I am certain that the others were similarly moved."[38]

Technically, the operation appeared to have worked perfectly, but eleven days later Gregory died from postoperative pneumonia. Conscious of the potential of artificial heart-lung machines to provide much longer time on bypass, Lillehei asked one of his research colleagues, Richard DeWall, to explore designing a less cumbersome version of Gibbon's device. A radical thinker, DeWall developed an entirely new type of machine called a bubble oxygenator, which was cheap, safe, and easy to assemble and sterilize. It revolutionized open-heart surgery. By mid-1956, DeWall and

Lillehei had used it to operate successfully on nearly a hundred patients. Word spread fast. Suddenly, teams all over America had the confidence to launch open-heart surgery programs of their own. Surgeons from across the world came to watch DeWall and Lillehei at work before disseminating their new techniques back at home. Nothing appeared to be off-limits. Thanks to the heart-lung machine, there was not a single type of heart disease that was not, at least in theory, amenable to surgical correction.

Some fifty years later, in 2004, Denton Cooley, surgeon-in-chief at the Texas Heart Institute, paid tribute to Lillehei's role as the "father of heart surgery," who had ushered in this dizzying new era of limitless potential for surgical incursions on the human heart: "The credit belongs to Lillehei and his colleagues for opening the door—for providing the key to an exciting era. At a medical meeting shortly after Lillehei's historic intracardiac operation, I said that he had provided 'the can opener to the biggest picnic cardiac surgeons had ever known.' Even now, I couldn't agree more."[39]

The most bewitching possibility of all was lost to no one, not least an ambitious young surgical trainee from South Africa who had heard about the incredible work of a group of pioneering heart surgeons in Minnesota, and applied to join Lillehei's team. When Christiaan Barnard first set eyes on the heart-lung machine being used by Lillehei during open-heart surgery in 1955, he was intoxicated:

Even now I can recall the details of that morning, the first time I witnessed the life of a human being held in a coil of plastic tubes and a whirling pump. This was more than a machine. It was the gateway to surgery beyond anything yet known. While it stood in for heart and lungs, vast repairs could be made inside the body. New valves could be put inside the heart, maybe even a whole heart itself.[40]

———

Max sat cradled in his father's lap, clutching a cuddly monkey that wore its own miniature surgical mask to keep him company as he went into theater. High as a shooting star on his pre-meds, he swung wildly from tears to peals of ecstatic laughter. Emma and Paul donned their own surgical gowns to accompany their son into theater. The anesthesiologist and a member of the surgical team performed a comedy routine with glove puppets to distract him as Max was wheeled inside. The lights were so bright they hurt Paul's eyes. He saw a huge table, its contents masked by multiple towels, under which, he knew, an armory of surgical instruments lay hidden. He saw the heart-lung machine, its vast coils of tubing and wire and complexity, a chaotic caricature of a human heart and lungs. He saw the banks of monitors and infusions and pumps with which every inch of the theater was festooned. All of it alien, otherworldly, wrong: a theater more suited to an astronaut than a child. And then there was Max. Tiny, whimpering, his white-blond hair soaked with sweat as his parents endeavored to calm him.

It was four o'clock in the afternoon. Before he pressed down a syringe, the anesthesiologist told Max to try to stay awake as long as he could. "Why do I feel so sleepy?" Max asked, and a moment later fell unconscious. Paul and Emma bent down to kiss him. "As I lifted my face away from his, I couldn't help it," Paul says. "Our son was about to have major open-heart surgery and we had been told he had a twenty percent chance of not making it. I turned and burst into tears. I may have just had my last kiss with my son, seen him alive for the last time, and the emotion was all-consuming. I had never felt anything like it before. My insides were being wrenched and I was suffocating."

Matching

Just before 9 a.m. on Tuesday, August 1, 2017, Joe Ball meets a specialist nurse in organ donation named Vanessa Pritchard. Nurses like Vanessa are highly trained in how to introduce the topic of donation gently and delicately, with all the sensitivity a family's grief and pain demands. On this occasion, none of that tact is necessary. Joe and his daughters, Keely and Katelyn, decided the night before that Keira, without question, would have wanted to help others through donating her organs. Not only has the decision already been made, but Katelyn and Keely are overflowing with pride that their little sister can do something so extraordinary at the end of her life. "I walked into a very calm room where Katelyn was painting Keira's nails orange," says Vanessa. "It felt so peaceful, as though they'd already accepted that Keira was likely to be dead at that point. We know that's the shock, we know it hasn't fully hit them yet. But they were just pushing ahead. When we talked about organ donation, Joe said it was obvious. There was no back-and-forth, no worries, nothing they wanted me to explain further. Joe just said, 'Absolutely, this is exactly what she would have wanted. We are totally confident about that and so we want the same.' We did all the paperwork there and then, even before the neurological death testing."

Inside Keira's cubicle in the PICU, something subtle yet foundational has shifted. Prior to this moment, there has been no good news. The hypotheticals have formed a litany of loss: What if she never wakes up, what if she never speaks or laughs again, what if, even as we watch the rise and fall of her chest, she has already died and is no longer here with us? Now, for the first time, there is something beyond the bleakness of these four blank walls. The present is infused with possibility.

Away from Joe and his daughters, Vanessa's phone calls and emails start a chain reaction, spurring others into action who, in turn, stir others to act. A PICU consultant must inform the coroner that a family wishes for their relative to become an organ donor. The coroner must give their consent for organ retrieval. The police need to be involved—as a road traffic casualty, Keira will likely require a forensic postmortem. Joe and the PICU team need to talk to Loanna, Keira's mother, who is recovering from major surgery to her shattered limbs in the adult ICU of an adjacent hospital. The GP must be contacted to supply details of Keira's entire past medical history. Blood must be taken and rushed to a laboratory to check for viruses, infections, anything that might preclude Keira becoming a donor. A second blood sample needs to be urgently couriered for tissue typing. All of it frantic, all of it *now*, because although Keira is as stable as her doctors can make her, her brain is so severely damaged that her body is at risk of sudden cardiovascular collapse.

Inside the cubicle, Keira's family is cocooned away from the fevered activity, and deliberately so. Her lead PICU nurse, Jemma Evans, is doing her utmost to ensure that the atmosphere is as conducive as possible to enable Joe and his children to cherish these hours with Keira. "It is such a privilege to care for a child and their family on intensive care, in that most difficult time in their life. You're a complete stranger to them, their child is very sick or even dying, and this family is giving you their trust. We are in a unique and very special position," she says. A play specialist contacts the PICU and arranges for Katelyn and Keely to join their brother, Bradley, who is recovering from major abdominal surgery on another ward. "She got them making friendship bracelets and I remember thinking at the time, 'What a fantastic idea.' They made one each for themselves and then one for Keira to wear, too, so they all matched. I thought to myself, 'this is something that is going to be able to go with Keira into theater when the time comes.' That's so powerful, isn't it?"

Shortly after three o'clock in the afternoon, the PICU consultant, Dr. Alvin Schadenberg, and his registrar arrive to perform the brain death testing. Jemma, an experienced ICU nurse, has anticipated this moment. "As soon as I'd come in on the Monday and seen what Keira's intracranial pressure and her scan results were, I knew that she was going to die. I didn't expect anything to change after the brain stem testing because I felt that she had already gone. Her body was alive, for sure, but that was because we were keeping her body alive. I treated her exactly as if she was alive, I mean, I talked to her the whole time. I would say, 'Oh, okay, I'm just going to move you there so you're a bit more comfortable,' or 'Let's just brush your hair,' or 'I just need to turn you a minute to care for you, so we need to gently turn you onto your side.' It is really, really important to keep doing that, even though you know they are almost certainly gone."

Everyone leaves the room apart from Joe and Katelyn, neither of whom can bear to leave Keira's side. Katelyn has multiple reasons for being determined to stay, no matter how distressing she finds the testing process. Most important, there is her fierce, protective loyalty: she could never abandon her little sister. Another, more clandestine motive is rooted in suspicion: she does not entirely trust these doctors and their doctors' talk. She will scrutinize them, hawklike, through every step of the testing, hoping through her vigilance to spot a response from Keira that has somehow passed the experts by. Those words that sit like lead on her chest—*irreversible, brain dead, already gone*—cannot be as absolute as the doctors maintain. If she does her job, if she just looks hard enough, surely she may yet save her sister. The line between what Katelyn knows to be true and what she wants to believe is beginning to buckle and fracture.

Clinical protocols for determining brain death are rigid, detailed, and followed to the letter. Crucially, they err on the side of life. If there is any doubt, ambiguity, or disagreement about the results, then the patient is presumed *not* to be brain dead. The tests must be performed by two different doctors in precisely the right way and precisely the right order. They are repeated to ensure that nothing about the first set of results is erroneous.[1] Each test tries to elicit a specific brain stem reflex. If even one of the reflexes can be elicited, then the patient cannot be said to be brain dead. But if *all* the reflexes are absent, then there is no longer any connection between the upper brain and the rest of the body. You are, officially, dead. Before testing can begin, any sedating drugs must be withdrawn so that there is no artificial suppression of the brain stem. So, too, must hypothermia, biochemical disturbances, low levels of oxygen, and high levels of carbon dioxide be corrected, in case they are contributing to the patient's unresponsiveness. In Keira's case, all sedation was stopped some thirty-six hours earlier. Since that time, nothing. Her comatose state—inert and unflinching, despite the endotracheal tube snaking from the ventilator into her lungs—is entirely due to her brain injuries. As Alvin Schadenberg prepares to begin testing, there is little doubt in his mind as to what the results will be.

With Joe and Katelyn following his every move, Alvin starts by shining a flashlight into Keira's eyes to see if they react to the light. The pupillary reflex should cause her pupils to constrict in response to the brightness. Instead, they remain fixed and dilated: they do not respond to the light at all. Next, Alvin leans in a little closer so that he can gently brush the surface of her eyeballs with cotton.

Ordinarily, this would trigger a corneal reflex—a blink or a wink as the patient involuntarily endeavors to protect their vision. Keira's eyelids, though, remain motionless. Now the testing becomes unavoidably invasive. In order to check for the vestibulo-ocular reflex, Alvin must squirt a syringe full of ice-cold water into one of Keira's ears. The cold should trigger a movement of her eyes toward the ear, but again, it elicits nothing. Testing the gag reflex is more invasive still. It entails placing a spatula at the back of the throat and seeing if the patient coughs or splutters. Keira, predictably, does neither.

The fact is, unlike the spinal reflexes with which most of us are familiar—the brisk lurch of the shin in response to a tap on the knee from a doctor's tendon hammer, for example—brain stem reflexes are the deepest, most primal responses we ever make to the world that surrounds us. Their testing is necessarily intimate, transgressive. Probing the ear and throat of a patient as they lie unconscious crosses boundaries and breaches bodily integrity. "Parts of the brain stem testing are not nice to watch," says Jemma. "They are not things you would ever usually do to a person or let someone else do. It's quite a strange thing to see. All the time we had been talking to Keira as though she was alive, being gentle with her, putting her in positions that looked normal and natural and comfortable. But now these were medical procedures happening to Keira. I suppose that was when the reality started to hit Joe."

The hardest test of all for a family to witness is the final one: the attempt to elicit spontaneous breathing. The only way to do so is to disconnect the patient from the ventilator and see what happens next. As time ticks by without a breath being drawn, carbon dioxide builds up in the bloodstream because it is not being expelled through the lungs. Ordinarily, high levels of carbon dioxide would be detected in the brain stem and trigger a breath. The absence of breathing is therefore another piece of evidence signifying brain death. The "apnea test" sounds straightforward when described objectively, but for a family, the minutes that elapse without a breath can be agony to endure. You wait and wait, silently willing the person whom you love to breathe, knowing you would give your own life to make it happen. "When we take a child off the ventilator and they don't breathe, for parents this is often the first moment of absolute clarity," says Jemma. "Until then, they've often looked like they're fine because they're on the ventilator. They look like they're breathing for themselves. But when you see that physically nothing is happening with the testing, you start to think, 'My child is not there because I can see she's not breathing.'"

For Joe, it is almost too painful to witness. He has now been in the PICU for forty-eight hours and he cannot take any more. When Alvin reconnects Keira to the ventilator—and only then does her chest resume its rise and fall—Joe leaves the cubicle in tears. It is 4:02 p.m. All of the tests must now be repeated by a different doctor—Alvin's registrar—but the conclusion has already been drawn. Nothing, and everything, has changed. Keira was one thing and now she is another. The doctors, with as much sensitivity as they can muster, shine the flashlight, pick up another wisp of cotton, and reach once more for the syringe of iced water. Katelyn refuses to move from her sister's side. The Earth still turns and Keira's heart still beats, but as Katelyn twists the braided orange cotton round and round her wrist, she has no words.

4:02 p.m.—the point at which the first complete set of brain stem tests failed to elicit any signs of life—is officially recorded as the time of Keira's death. Although her body appears to live on, the irreversible failure of the brain stem denotes the cessation of life. The moment marks a subtle shift in the manner of her care. If anything, the tenderness with which Jemma treats Keira is heightened, not diminished. Perhaps, in the face of all they have lost, this extra solicitude is a way of showing her family that everything she means to them still lives, is still loved, and that this is the only form of afterlife that counts. Jemma slips Keira's hospital gown from her shoulders and carefully reclothes her in her favorite pajamas, the soft Mickey Mouse ones with the silky buttons. She brushes her hair until it gleams on the pillow and tucks her toy puppy safely under her arm. "We wanted to take her home just as she was so we could keep on holding her," says Katelyn. "We were told she was brain dead, but she still looked perfect."

Even though her shift has already ended—and she has been at work for thirteen hours—Jemma stays on to attend to the matter of memory boxes, which can bring enormous comfort to grieving families. Usually, the PICU nurses help family members choose what they would like to put in them. Handprints, footprints, and locks of hair are common choices. Sometimes children like to put their own drawings of their sibling into the box. Parents will often keep a hospital wristband. For babies, the nurses can make casts or imprints of tiny hands and feet using a mold and plaster of Paris. "We always give a family in this situation a memory box with precious little things in it, but we're only supposed to give one per family," says Jemma. "I made four, one for each of Keira's siblings and one for Joe and Loanna. I had to restock the memory box supplies, but I just went online and bought some more supplies for the unit."

One person is absent from this painstaking curation of memories. Loanna remains heavily sedated in intensive care, too unwell to be involved. Although Keira's doctors have asked her permission to donate Keira's organs—and she was only too eager to grant it—this period of her life is destined to remain a blur, perhaps mercifully so.

Keira's nursing and medical team have a new clinical focus—that of optimizing her physiology so as to deliver donor organs in the best possible condition. The goal is no longer the resuscitation of an injured brain but the restoration of cardiac and lung function in order to preserve the health of her organs. Adhering meticulously to a detailed donor management protocol, the team addresses this task with the utmost gravity.[2] Anything else, arguably, would be a betrayal of the trust a donor family has placed in the people who proposed organ donation as a part of their loved one's end-of-life care. "Now that the hope was Keira would become an organ donor in the morning, we needed to concentrate very hard to ensure she remained in a stable condition," recalls Alvin. "As a medical team, your priority is to support a grieving family, but you also do everything you can to keep all the observations in the normal range, so that the organs are well perfused and stay in good condition." For the nursing team, this requires constant and meticulous juggling of multiple infusions of fluids and medications. "Until then, our sole focus had been caring for Keira," says Jemma, "but now, in a way, we were caring for other children, too, because parts of Keira were going to be retrieved and given to somebody else, and hopefully she was going to save their lives."

Shortly after 5 p.m., the coroner's office calls the hospital to confirm that permission for the removal of Keira's organs has been granted. Alvin immediately informs the hospital's operating theaters that a retrieval is likely. A theater is set aside for Keira for as long as it is needed. Everyone knows what pediatric retrieval means. This is the tragedy whose grace is its power to save, to avert other tragedies, to preserve other parents from this intolerable pain. No one questions, no one quibbles—the staff is galvanized to do anything required to help Keira save lives.

At eight o'clock that night, word reaches the PICU that Keira's tissue typing results are back. Of all the pieces of information being frantically assembled before her organs can be matched, this is one of the most critical. Tissue typing enables doctors to assess how compatible with a recipient an organ is likely to be. Put crudely, the more closely matched a donor organ and a recipient's tissues, the longer the recipient is likely to live. Like the wildly unsuitable boyfriend and girlfriend whose friends raise their eyebrows but keep their concerns to themselves, significantly mismatched donor and recipient tissues lead to painful, public, predictable rejection. Indeed, so effective is the body's immune system at identifying and attacking any hint of foreign invasion—be it bacterial, viral, or fungal—that even those patients with the best-matched organs face the lifelong threat of rejection. The most aggressive immuno-suppressant medications cannot necessarily stop the body turning on a transplanted organ, with potentially fatal results. It is for this reason that the person regarded by many modern transplant surgeons as the true hero of their specialty is neither a surgeon, nor even a doctor. Peter Medawar's dazzling contribution to the field was inspired one sunny afternoon during the Second World War when a man, quite literally, fell burning from the sky.

———

Peter Medawar was lazing in his North Oxford garden with his wife and daughter when a roar from above caused them to tilt their heads skyward. "We saw a huge two-engined bomber approaching us over the housetops," he recalls in his autobiography.[3] The British aircraft, probably en route to RAF Brize Norton, was in distress and crashed into the garden of another house a mere two hundred yards from where the Medawars were sitting. The moment would become an epiphany that defined the rest of Peter Medawar's life: "A scientist who wants to do something original and important must experience, as I did, some kind of shock that forces upon his intention the kind of problem that it should be his duty, and will become his pleasure, to investigate."

Until that fateful Sunday afternoon, Medawar regarded him-self as something of an academic dilettante. Described by one colleague as "abnormally handsome, hypnotically articulate in public,"[4] Medawar had studied zoology at Oxford as an undergraduate. Now a laboratory scientist in his mid-twenties, he feared that his postgraduate research to date had been an essentially fruitless endeavor. An academic supervisor responded to one of Medawar's ideas for a research project with the scathing line: "That would be quite a nice little experiment, wouldn't it, and that's what you really like, isn't it—little experiments?"[5] The turning point for Medawar came when a severely burned young airman was dragged alive from the wreckage of the bomber he had just witnessed plummeting to Earth. The airman was rushed to Oxford's Radcliffe Infirmary with 60 percent of the surface area of his body destroyed by full-thickness, third-degree burns. One of the clinicians caring for the airman, Dr. John Barnes, happened to be Medawar's research colleague in the university's pathology department. He urged Medawar to set aside his intellectual pursuits and come and visit the patient in order to try to devise practical suggestions that might help save his life.

At the time, the treatment of deep and extensive burns was in its infancy. As Medawar says, "In the old days the victims of such burns did not really raise a medical problem at all—they simply died—but by the outbreak of war the blood transfusion service was already on a firm footing and the sulfonamide drugs had been introduced, thus putting it in our power to combat the two principal causes of mortality after burning: loss of body fluid and wound infection."[6] Thanks to antibiotics and blood transfusions, by the early 1940s a severely burned patient could be kept alive through the acute stages of the burn. Then—at least in theory—the dead tissues would be sloughed off by the body, and skin grafts could be applied in their place. But doctors had learned from bitter experience that skin from another human being would not "take" as a permanent graft, save for in the exceptional circumstances of two people who happened to be identical twins. For everyone else, grafted skin from a donor would be rejected, withering and dying in a matter of days.

After meeting the stricken airman, Medawar focused his prodigious intellect on the challenge of finding a way of eking out what could be spared of the skin left on the patient's own body, so as to make one piece cover the area of three or four. He borrowed bits of leftover skin from the groundbreaking facial reconstructions being conducted in wartime by the plastic surgeon Sir Harold Gillies, using them to create a thin gruel of epidermal cells suspended in tissue culture that he termed "a kind of living skin soup."[7] He tried freezing human skin to minus 70 degrees Celsius, then carving it into slices a tiny fraction of an inch thick that were applied with a fine paintbrush to the area needing covering. Nothing worked. Although the airman survived, it was not thanks to Medawar's experiments but to a primitive "postage stamp" technique invented by a Spanish plastic surgeon.

Nevertheless, Medawar was hooked. He knew that if he could find a way to use homografts—skin transplanted from relatives or from other voluntary donors—without them being rejected, then the treatment of burn victims could be transformed. The fundamental mystery lay not in the clinical application but in the basic, underlying science. *How* did the body discriminate between its own and other living cells? *How* was it able to recognize "self" and "non-self" substances, ferociously attacking the latter, while permitting the former to flourish? If Medawar could unlock this secret, then the human body could potentially be manipulated through drugs, radiation, or some other means to enable homografts to take.

Medawar was consumed with the challenge of finding an answer. Rather than wasting any more time castigating himself for the years he had previously frittered away (as he saw it), he successfully applied to the War Wounds Committee of the UK Medical Research Council for funding to investigate the problem. Moving to the Burns Unit of Glasgow Royal Infirmary in Scotland, he teamed up with a Scottish surgeon named Tom Gibson to try and see with his own eyes exactly what happened to skin homografts that differentiated them from autografts (grafted skin from the patient's own body). A hospital inpatient with extensive third-degree burns from her gas fire, "Mrs. McK," allowed the pair to graft on her a small population of homografts from a donor, as well as a population of autografts taken from elsewhere on her body. Each sliver of skin was approximately a quarter of an inch in diameter. At regular intervals, they removed one graft from each population to examine under a microscope what was happening to it. Initially, all the grafts seemed to take. But after a few days, the homografts were being visibly invaded by a particular kind of white blood cell known as a lymphocyte, and subsequently destroyed. Next, the pair applied a second set of homografts to Mrs. McK. This time, the grafts were set upon and destroyed almost immediately. It was as though the body's initial response to the foreign tissue had somehow primed the lymphocytes to mount a quicker and deadlier response the second time round.

In 1943, Medawar and Gibson published their seminal paper, "The Fate of Skin Homografts in Man."[8] Based on their findings with Mrs. McK, who was well enough to be discharged from hospital a month after the experimental grafting, the authors presented the hypothesis that skin homografts were rejected by the same kind of immunological process that eliminates unwanted bacteria and viruses from the body. Somehow, the immune system treated homografts in the same way as it did these foreign organisms, aggressively targeting them with lymphocytes. Crucial to their theory was the idea that this response was not "innate" but "adaptive"—in other words, rather than being a built-in response that Mrs. McK had been born with, it was one that had evolved each time she encountered the homografts. The accelerated destruction of the second set of homografts was the key piece of evidence for this view. When Medawar returned to Oxford, he set about corroborating his findings by systematically studying the phenomenon of homograft rejection in laboratory animals—primarily several hundred rabbits. Lacking any support in the form of trained technicians, he not only cut, stained, and photographed thousands of microscopic sections himself, he also fed, watered, and mucked out the cages of his subjects, publishing two papers on the fate of skin homografts in rabbits in 1944.

In the immediate postwar years, it was not exactly clear how any of this would lessen the formidable challenges faced by surgeons eager to transplant human organs. All such attempts to date had ended in abject failure. The organ would be stitched into place, die rapidly, and no one understood why. At the turn of the century, Alexis Carrel, the French surgeon responsible for developing the technique of vascular anastomosis, had referred to a mysterious "biological force" that somehow destroyed transplanted organs, while being oblivious as to what that force entailed.[9] Medawar's proposition—that it was the immune system rejecting foreign tissues—led scientists in the early 1950s to attempt to prolong the life of skin grafts in animals by aggressively weakening the recipient's immune system. Unfortunately, the methods tried—total body irradiation or fearsomely potent steroids—had an exceedingly narrow "therapeutic window," meaning that the doses needed to keep the graft alive had a frustrating tendency to kill the recipient.[10] There was simply no margin of safety and many doctors at the time felt nihilistic about the future of transplantation.

Then, in 1951, Medawar changed everything. He embarked on a series of experiments that would culminate in the paper that earned him a Nobel Prize and that led Thomas Starzl—the American surgeon responsible for transplanting the first-ever human liver—to describe him as a medical Galileo, the sixteenth-century astronomer who famously championed the radical view that the sun, not the Earth, was the center of the universe: "Armed with dissecting scissors, a few rabbits and mice in a dilapidated London laboratory . . . [Medawar] founded a new field that crossed all specialty barriers and blurred, as no-one ever had before, the distinction between basic and clinical science."[11] Together with two colleagues, Rupert Billingham and Leslie Brent, Medawar set out to test a hypothesis proposed by an Australian immunologist, Frank Macfarlane Burnet. Burnet suspected that if foreign cells were introduced into an animal with a very immature immune system while it was still developing in utero, then as the animal matured, it would not reject future grafts from that source. Medawar and his team injected embryonic mice with cells from another mouse. When the mice matured, the team found they would accept skin and other tissues from the donor mouse, but not from any other mouse strain. They had developed, in short, "acquired immunologic tolerance" to foreign grafts—the first time anyone had demonstrated that such a phenomenon was possible.

Medawar's three-page paper, published in *Nature* in 1953,[12] so electrified the transplant community that Thomas Starzl described it as a "blinding beacon of hope."[13] He had shown it could be done. And if mice could be induced to tolerate foreign tissues, then why not humans, too? For the first time, clinicians' hopes were raised that there might be ways of inducing a kind of immunological insouciance in the recipients of transplanted organs that would prevent them from rejecting their grafts. Drugs that induced immunological tolerance without killing the patient no longer felt like science fiction but plausible reality. For their extraordinary contributions to the field of transplant medicine, Peter Medawar and Frank Macfarlane Burnet shared the 1960 Nobel Prize in medicine. Thomas

Starzl would later reflect that "most of the surgical specialties can be tracked to the creative vision of a surgeon. Transplantation is an exception. Here, the father of the field is succinctly defined in the dictionary as: 'Peter Brian Medawar.'"[14]

———

Tucked behind a large Sainsbury's supermarket and a nondescript retail park just off the Bristol ring road is a squat building that most people scarcely notice. Its flesh-colored bricks, olive-green paintwork, and dark concrete roof, flecked with moss and lichen, suggest nothing of particular note inside. The corridors within are equally drab. Low ceilings, dingy carpets, and little natural light. One hallway extends into an open-plan office containing twelve desks, each with a worn-out computer on top. In these decidedly humdrum surroundings, at exactly ten minutes to midnight on August 1, 2017, a chain of events begins with the potential to end in wonder. A telephone rings. The on-call specialist nurse in organ donation at the Bristol Royal Hospital for Children is on the line. Her exhaustive information-gathering, investigating, double-checking, and data-entering are, at last, complete. She is calling formally to register nine-year-old Keira Ball as a donor whose organs are ready to be listed and matched.

The NHS Blood and Transplant list is a living, breathing entity, organic and in flux from minute to minute, hour to hour. It comprises every person in the UK who wishes to have a transplant, who has been judged suitable to be listed, and in whom an organ is failing so badly that it imperils their life. The list is subdivided into organ-specific lists, each of which—heart, lung, liver, kidney, intestine, stomach, pancreas—is further subdivided into adult and pediatric lists. Due to the perennial shortage of child donors, pediatric lists crawl at the most glacial pace of all, causing immense anxiety for waiting parents. At any one time in the UK, around seven thousand people sit on the combined transplant waiting list. Of these, around four hundred die every year while waiting for a transplant.[15] In the US, the statistics are even more sobering. There are over one hundred thousand men, women, and children on the national transplant list, of whom seventeen die every day while waiting.[16]

It is completely by chance that the UK's national NHS Organ Donation and Transplant Hub happens to be situated in Bristol, the location of Keira's hospital. The center may be somewhat careworn, but when it comes to matching organs with patients, gleaming facades and ostentatious branding are not what count. Military-grade logistics and highly motivated teams are what really make the difference, and under the leadership of the head of hub operations, Michael Stokes, both abound. Upon leaving the army in 2012 after two decades of service, Michael was intrigued by a recruitment advertisement he spotted for organ retrieval. When it became apparent, mid-interview, that the transplant service was not in fact looking for couriers but for logistical expertise, Michael swiftly recalibrated his mental image of driving at speed across the UK with precious cargoes of human hearts in the back of his car. He started as a shift manager and rose rapidly through the ranks to lead the service by 2016. At any moment, night or day, a team of five or six coordinators, led by a shift manager, is responsible for managing and coordinating the offers of all donor organs in the UK. "The throughput these days is incredible," says Michael. "The numbers of potential donors used to be small, but now, in any twenty-four-hour period, we probably get about forty to sixty referral calls from hospitals about possible donors that all need to be assessed and triaged. Those referrals end up in about eight to ten actual donors on average every twenty-four hours."

That night, a coordinator enters Keira's age, height, weight, blood group, and tissue type into the national donor database. A second coordinator cross-checks the data independently: human error in record-ing these vital facts could be calamitous. Next, the coordinator assigns an ID number to Keira to ensure her anonymity. From this moment on, in every exchange between the hub and the various hospitals who may be offered her organs, Keira exists only in code. With a resource as precious and scarce as organs, it is essential to strip sentiment out of the matching process to ensure it is as equitable as possible. Fairness dictates that the distribution of organs should be formulaic, governed not by human emotions but hard utilitarian logic. Accordingly, a com-puter algorithm generates the lists of matches, based entirely on how likely an organ is to survive in each recipient on the list, given their size, age, blood group, and tissue type.

Every person waiting on the list helps to refine future iterations of the algorithm by providing real-time-outcomes data that is fed back into the model. For the rest of their lives, whether they receive an organ, languish or flourish, experience rejection, live or die, that information will be codified, quantified, and added to the evidence base upon which new organs are allocated. Like grains of sand, the tiniest details of each person's blood tests, echocardiograms, medication changes, and general health combine to build the bed-rock upon which future lives depend. Geography is crucial, too, particularly for heart transplants. Evidence shows that even when enveloped in a bed of ice, hearts can only withstand a few hours of "cold ischemic time" before the tissue may become irreparably damaged.[17] Ideally no more than four hours should elapse between the removal of a heart and its implantation into a recipient's chest. The pediatric heart transplant list is therefore subdivided into three categories: super-urgent, urgent, and non-urgent. The first match-ing run takes place against the small number of cases whose need is super-urgent. These are the children whose hearts are so spent they could die from one moment to the next.

Briefly, the coordinator's finger hovers above the keyboard. The algorithm means that launching a matching run is both momentous and peculiarly banal. With one click of a mouse, the algorithm fires, and after two or three minutes of permutations, a ranked list of matches begins to fill the monitor. Matters of life and death, in Excel spreadsheet form. The coordinator knows that the list of names she is about to generate will thud into the world like a mortal decree, a life-and-death diktat, plucking one child from the abyss while condemning others to remain on the precipice. It is extraordinary, godlike, terrifying. Click, run. Click, run. Super-urgent, urgent, non-urgent. The printer whirs and the sheets of paper flop out.

There are thirteen children in need of urgent or super-urgent heart transplants who match Keira's size and blood group. The child at the top of the list is the same age as Keira, nine years old. His name is Max Johnson.

Waiting

Seven and a half hours after leaving Max unconscious on an operating table, Emma and Paul could not bear the wait any longer. They picked up a phone and called the pediatric intensive care unit, desperate for an update on his open-heart surgery. "I'm glad you rang," said the nurse who answered, "because I was just about to call you. Max is being tidied up in theater and then he'll be on his way to a bed here. You can come on over." A single thought flowed like cognac through Paul. "He's made it. Max has made it. He's survived."

The titanium and gold HeartWare left ventricular assist device (LVAD) that Fabrizio De Rita had successfully stitched into the wall of Max's heart was whirring at three thousand revolutions per minute, expelling a continuous jet of blood from his left ventricle through a small plastic tube before returning it, under pressure, to his aorta. Max now had a "bridge to transplant"—a means of temporarily maintaining something close to a normal blood circulation while he waited for a suitable heart. For the first time in many months, his body was being steeped in properly oxygenated blood. Though he had no pulse—and would never regain one unless a matching donor heart could be found—his new blood pressure should revitalize his body. Fabrizio told Paul and Emma that the surgery had gone exactly as hoped. Unremarkably, in fact—the most coveted word in the realm of surgery, where excitement is the last thing a patient wishes to generate. "I remember shaking Fabrizio's hand and seeing how incredibly tired he was, but also how engaged," says Paul. "He seemed to really care about being able to give us this good news. I think it genuinely mattered to him."

Post-operation, Max was draped in so many wires, drains, tubes, and electrodes that it was hard to make out the boy buried beneath them. Only the glimpse of white-blond hair gave his identity away. "I remember saying something like 'Oh my God, look at all the wires,'" recalls Emma. "Nothing had prepared me for this. I had it in my head that we'd go in and he'd almost be sitting up with a plaster over his chest, but he had this huge dressing that went all the way down to his stomach where they'd opened him up. He looked so small, he was so very thin by then. There was nothing of him, he was just tubes and wires. His hair looked all dirty, like it needed a good wash and a comb. And the worst thing was, he was naked apart from this nappy. They'd had to put him in a nappy and it was like he'd regressed to being a baby. I just couldn't take it in." Observing the horrified look on Emma's face, one of the nurses reached out and gently rubbed her back in sympathy.

Max was deeply sedated and intubated, with a ventilator controlling his breathing. A wire now pierced his upper abdomen, traveling inside his chest cavity to the LVAD embedded deep within his heart. Externally, the wire ran to the battery packs and laptop computer with which the parameters of the LVAD were set and monitored. Max's life now relied essentially on being plugged into the mains. "He was so dependent on technology," says Paul. "If the LVAD stopped working, his heart would stop beating. But the thing that struck me most of all was his eyes. They were half-open and just looked completely vacant. It was like there was nothing there."

When Emma was invited to hold Max, she was almost too frightened to do it. "They moved him from the bed, saying, 'I'm sure you want to cuddle him,' and they lifted him up and put him on my lap, but I was worried stiff that I would knock one of the wires away or do something that could harm him. It was like holding a baby because he had the nappy on, but he was too big to be a baby. I remember his legs just flopping down over mine and not feeling comfortable at all because I was so scared. I wanted him back in his bed so he would be safe." Paul and Emma only stayed with Max for a handful of shell-shocked minutes. It was abundantly clear he needed the expert nursing of the PICU team far more than anything they could offer. As they walked back to their accommodation, neither of them quite knew how to articulate the trauma of what they had just witnessed. "We just shared a look," says Paul, "that expressed something like 'Oh my God. How the hell did we get here? How did this happen? How has our healthy little boy reached this point?'"

The unnerving odds that Max had faced on the table—Paul was told he had a one-in-five chance of not surviving the surgery—had at least arisen within the context of heart surgeons having amassed over half a century of experience in implanting LVADs. There was nothing experimental about Max's procedure, which was perilous primarily because of his heightened risk of a cardiac arrest. The first patient in whom an LVAD was successfully implanted, on the other hand, was in essence a human laboratory. In 1966, when the ground-breaking surgery took place, it had only been attempted once before in a human, with the patient never regaining consciousness.[1] Yet when Michael DeBakey, a pioneering American cardiac surgeon, confronted the crisis unfolding on the table before him, he reasoned, quite rightly, that his patient had nothing to lose.

Today, as then, DeBakey is regarded as one of the giants of 1960s cardiac surgery, whose surgical talent and ferocious productivity are matched only by his fearsome reputation. In his book *Open Heart: The Radical Surgeons Who Revolutionized Medicine*, the transplant surgeon David Cooper, himself a surgical trainee in the 1960s, notes with awe the 60,000 operations personally performed by DeBakey, not to mention his 1,500 published papers.[2] DeBakey attributed his prodigious output to his steely will and a seemingly superhuman disregard for sleep: "You know that you have a certain time span, whatever God gives you. When you are living, you want to enjoy that. When you are sleeping, you are just dead as far as conscious living is concerned; that's part of your death. So I think you have to set some goals and priorities. I try to use my time as efficiently as I can."[3] That expectation extended to everyone on DeBakey's team, but with particular ruthlessness to his surgical residents. One of them, Bud Frazier, describes how the residents would be "horrified" as DeBakey tore strips off them for incompetence, sloth, and downright stupidity. He demanded life-and-soul devotion to the job at hand:

> Dr. DeBakey wouldn't let you leave the hospital. As a resident, you were in the ICU for 90 days at a stretch. You were not allowed out of the hospital at all for 90 days—unless you were fired, that was the only way you could get out. You were not allowed to leave the ICU during this period, not even to go to the hospital cafeteria; food was brought up to you. You slept in the ICU. If you were married, your wife and kids could only see you if they came to the ICU.[4]

On August 8, 1966, DeBakey had spent four hours performing open-heart surgery on a thirty-seven-year-old woman to replace—successfully—two damaged valves in her heart. When it came, however, to disconnecting her from the heart-lung machine, he discovered that the shock of the surgery had stunned her heart, leaving it incapable of beating independently.[5] She faced two options: immediate death on the table or an unproven, speculative attempt to sew an artificial pump, the LVAD, into her heart, hoping it would act as a temporary bridge to the point at which her heart regained its function. Having honed his technique in the laboratory on scores of dogs, DeBakey reasoned that a slim possibility of saving his patient's life was better than no chance at all. Happily, the gamble paid off. For the next ten days, the LVAD performed the hard labor of pumping blood throughout the woman's body, giving her own heart a chance to heal. It was then removed, and the patient made a perfect recovery.

DeBakey's achievement epitomized the new era of open-heart surgery ushered in by heart-lung machines in the late 1950s and '60s. Cardiac surgeons, galvanized by the chance to write their name for posterity across a blank surgical canvas, rushed to test the limits of what their specialty could achieve—secretly hoping, perhaps, to win the coveted prize of achieving a historic surgical milestone of their own. The romance of the race to be first to stake a claim to new territory was seized upon by journalists at the time, who found themselves drawn to these derring-do tales of surgical heroes with pluck, guts, and bristling machismo (they were, without exception, men). In 1957, for example, *Time* magazine ran a ten-page feature on heart surgery with a surgeon, Charles Bailey, immortalized on the cover under the headline "Surgery's New Frontier."[6] The article celebrated the transformation of cardiac surgery from a "blunt, blind art" into a maestro-led endeavor with sufficient finesse to "approach the center of life itself." Its practitioners' willingness to experiment on patients was framed not as reckless but as commendably brave, for the fainthearted would never "push the limits set by Nature." The piece concluded prophetically: "Bailey refuses to believe there are no more conquests ahead. As he sees it, nothing is impossible in surgery. Bailey looks forward to the day when an entire heart may be taken from a man killed in an accident and grafted into another whose heart is diseased. Fantastic? 'Merely a matter of time,' says Surgeon Bailey."

Some of the heart surgeons of the era seem almost to have reveled in the media's depiction of their profession as a class of superhuman outliers with exceptional gifts and unmatchable courage. Perhaps they were seduced by the other great race of the decade—to deploy science, technology, daring, and tenacity to put a man on the moon. Boundless ambition was evidently seen as another prerequisite for success. For example, in a second *Time* cover story celebrating surgery in 1963, one of the surgeons interviewed gave his opinion as to which qualities were essential for becoming a great surgeon: "To be great . . . a surgeon must have a fierce determination to be the leader in his field. He must have a driving ego. A hunger beyond money. He must have a passion for perfectionism. He is like the actor who wants his name in lights."[7] The article drew a reverential parallel between the space race and surgical endeavor: "Man may strain ever farther into space, ever deeper into the heart of the atom, but there in the operating room all the results of the most improbable reaches of research, all the immense accumulation of medical knowledge, are drawn upon in a determined drive toward the most awesome goal of all: the preservation of one human life." Framed in this way, the human body, like the dark side of the moon, was merely a foreign territory, passively waiting to be colonized. Patients' hearts were there to be conquered.

Beneath the hyperbolic press coverage, genuine reasons for excitement abounded during the golden era of heart surgery. If not quite the medical equivalent of the first astronauts—not least because the only lives ever being put at risk were those of their patients, not their own—the pioneers of open-heart surgery invented, then refined, innovative techniques at a dazzling rate. More than any other surgeon, the person responsible for advancing heart transplantation from a state of wild speculation into sober reality was a mild-mannered and modest individual, Norman Shumway, chief of cardiothoracic surgery at Stanford University in California.[8] Shumway moved to Stanford after training in Minnesota under the great Clarence Walton Lillehei, the heart surgeon who had established conclusively the safety of open-heart surgery on a heart-lung machine in the mid-1950s. Working alongside his friend and colleague Richard Lower, Shumway conducted experimental studies on dogs for over a decade before he considered it responsible and, indeed, ethical to try to transplant a heart into a human. The reason the pair had first attempted to transplant a canine heart was not in order to pursue future glory but simply to alleviate boredom: they were embroiled in a particularly protracted experimental surgery during which they had nothing better to do.[9]

At the time, Shumway and Lower were investigating how long a heart could survive without damage when cut off from warm, oxygenated blood and bathed instead in icy saline. The aim of the technique, which they called topical hypothermia, was to stop the heart beating, create a bloodless operating field, and reduce the metabolic demands of the heart, perhaps even for as long as an hour before it would need to be reconnected to its supply of blood and oxygen. This would, they hoped, be of great clinical benefit, giving surgeons valuable extra time in which to operate safely on an opened heart.[10]

The pair soon discovered that a dog's heart could comfortably tolerate upward of an hour of topical hypothermia.[11] Once they had opened the chest of a dog, connected it to a heart-lung machine, and clamped the aorta and vena cava, there was nothing to do for the next sixty minutes except stare at a cold limp canine heart sitting motionless in a tub of brine. But nothing infuriates a surgeon more than being forced to twiddle their thumbs during a surgery. So, one day, unable to bear the dawdling any longer, Shumway and Lower decided to fill the hiatus by polishing their surgical skills. They would cut the dog's heart free from its moorings, removing it from the chest cavity, and then reattach it again—all during the hour of experimental cooling. To their surprise, they found it wasn't terribly difficult to do, so in subsequent cases they decided to raise the stakes by implanting not the original heart but that of *another* anesthetized dog. They knew the immune system would reject the transplanted organ eventually, but what would happen in the interim? They were astonished to discover that the dogs with transplanted hearts would be up and about, sniffing blithely round the laboratory, a mere twenty-four hours after their surgery. Without any immunosuppression, the dogs survived for anything from three days to almost three weeks, depending on the degree of tissue compatibility.[12]

Shumway and Lower did not stop there. As well as perfecting the operative technique for a heart transplant, they experimented with immunosuppressive regimes to prolong the survival of the transplanted hearts. They discovered that they could reverse an episode of acute rejection with the right combination of drugs and, crucially, that when rejection was occurring, it was accompanied by distinctive ECG changes.[13] This enabled the pair to diagnose rejection and give powerful immunosuppressants only when needed, meaning that the dogs were less vulnerable to serious infections.[14] The duo were grappling, in essence, with what is still today the single greatest challenge in transplant medicine—how to tune down the immune system just enough so that a transplant will take, yet not so much that the patient is defenseless against infectious diseases. Their painstaking juggling of rejection and infection enabled them to achieve remarkable long-term survival rates in dogs of over a year post-transplant.[15]

Finally, in November 1967, after ten years of research during which he had transplanted the hearts of more than three hundred dogs, Shumway believed he had sufficient clinical expertise in managing rejection to justify attempting to transplant a human heart. On November 20, he announced that he was ready to carry out the first human heart transplant and was awaiting a suitable donor.[16] The news coverage swept round the world. But thirteen days later, to widespread consternation in the field of cardiac surgery, the bombshell news broke that the man who had taken the final step of turning heart transplantation from veterinary experiment into human therapy was not, in fact, Norman Shumway, but the leader of a small surgical team in apartheid South Africa. The surgeon in question, Christiaan Barnard, had been quietly and stealthily competing for years to win the crown of achieving the world's first heart transplant.

———

Initially, the effect of Max's LVAD was transformative. He no longer spent his days curled up in bed with a painful swollen liver, but found he had the energy to walk, build Legos, and play pranks on the nurses. The parts of his body that had been chronically impaired by lack of oxygen, sluggishly existing, started to function with renewed vigor. He put on weight, his cheeks brightened, and he found he could concentrate on small chunks of schoolwork. For a while, waiting on the transplant list seemed entirely manageable. But the improvement was short-lived. As weeks turned into months with no news of a donor heart, Max's optimism began to dwindle. The nurses did their utmost to rally his spirits. Sometimes, at the end of a thirteen-hour shift, one of them would drive the seven-mile round trip to McDonald's to buy him, at their own expense, a bag of his favorite french fries. On her days off, Faye, a nurse whom Max adored, used to deliberately walk her German shepherd dog, Sydney, in the park beside the hospital so that Max could join them in his wheelchair, being pushed at high speed until he giggled with glee.

"The nurses were absolutely amazing," says Paul. "Their kindness and professionalism were just exceptional." But the longer Max languished in bed, too weak and breathless to walk, the more depressed he became.

Unbeknownst to anyone at this time, he recorded a video on his mobile phone in which he spoke directly into the camera. His face looks deathly pale with sunken eyes, the features contorted by anger and tears. Above the noise of nurses laughing somewhere on the ward behind him, Max can be heard saying, "I hate my life. I *hate* my life. I'm going to commit suicide when my dad comes back. I'm going to make myself dead." At nine years old, his months on the transplant list had been so traumatic he was not merely experiencing suicidal thoughts, he had decided to enact them. His doctors were baffled when, a few days later, he developed a raging temperature. They managed to isolate the source of his infection to the wires running from the LVAD embedded in the wall of his heart out of the skin of his abdomen. Only many months later, once home from his transplant, would Max show Emma the video recording, confessing that *he* had been the cause of the infection. His life had become so intolerable that he had tried to wrench out the wires connecting his LVAD to its battery pack, hoping his heart would stop beating. Had he been successful, he might easily have died. As it was, the damage he had caused to the skin around the wires created a portal for infection that could also have been deadly.

Paul's and Emma's lives were on hold, too, with unrelenting stress and no end in sight. "Waiting on the transplant list had begun to feel like being on death row. It was torture, purgatory, highly emotional, and both physically and mentally draining," says Paul. One day, Emma was walking past the Children's Heart Unit Fund charity shop when she came across the mother of another child on the ward, crouched on the floor and howling with such violence the sound seemed more animal than human. "Has some-thing happened?" Emma asked quietly. "She's gone," the mother screamed, referring to her daughter. A little girl, younger than Max, had just died on the ICU from complications of her recent transplant. A nurse appeared at a run to guide the mother to some privacy, leaving Emma poleaxed in her wake.

Around this time, Emma was approached by a journalist from the *Mirror* named Jeremy Armstrong. Jeremy happened to be friends with Andrew Leadbitter, the manager of the charitable accommodation for parents, Scott House, in which Emma and Paul were fortunate enough to have a room. Jeremy and Andrew had been chatting about a campaign that the *Mirror* had been running for three years entitled "Change the Law for Life." The aim of the campaign was simple: to persuade the government to change the law governing organ donation from an "opt in" to an "opt out" system, meaning that a person would be assumed to have given consent to donation unless they proactively stated otherwise. Someone's family would always have the right to overrule a dona-tion, but the hope was that the legal change would nevertheless lead to many more organs becoming available for transplant—and thus to many more lives like Max's being saved. Andrew knew how long Max had been waiting for a transplant and wondered whether his parents might consider speaking to Jeremy.

Paul and Emma agonized over whether to agree to speak to the *Mirror*. "We were very tentative to begin with, but the thought of being able to help change the law in a way that would help other people in the same awful situation as ours made us think, 'Okay, let's go for it,'" says Emma. "In a world where we had no control over Max's health, this was something where we could actively contrib-ute. We couldn't influence Max's health, but we could influence this. Being involved gave us a sense of purpose." They also knew that by sharing Max's story, they might just strike a chord with a bereaved family who would choose to consent to organ donation. They might, in other words, increase Max's chances of receiving a heart. "We understood the power of the media and we would do anything, if there was the slightest chance that Max would be saved. We also felt that if we didn't share Max's story, and if Max didn't make it in time for a new heart, that we would always regret not getting behind the campaign and potentially making a difference," says Paul.

In late June 2017, a photo of Max taken in the days after his LVAD surgery filled the entire front page of the *Mirror* beneath a headline that read "Our Plea to Theresa May—Change the Law for Max."[17] Beneath his white-blond hair, Max's eyes were huge and beseeching. A faint half smile played on his lips, which, like the rest of his face, were ghostly pale. His chest, bisected by a livid scar, was still stained with coppery iodine. There could not have been a more plaintive image of the hope and pain of a child's wait for a donor organ. Thousands of people were inspired by Max's story to sign a petition, organized by the *Mirror,* to change the law. At times, Emma and Paul found themselves feeling overwhelmed by the sheer number of friends and acquaintances who contacted them to say they had seen the article. Max's angelic features would appear on the newspaper's front page over and over again. The pressure on Prime Minister Theresa May was building.

Goodbye

It is precisely one minute past midnight. Inside the national NHS Organ Donation and Transplant Hub in Bristol, a coordinator has just called the Freeman Hospital in Newcastle to formally offer Keira's heart to Max. She has given the hospital one hour in which to decide whether to accept it. After that, she will offer it elsewhere. She will also call Great Ormond Street Hospital in London to make backup offers to the second and third most closely matched children after Max. A donor organ is far too precious to squander, so provisional offers are always made in case the first institution chooses to decline it.

In this case, there is no doubt at all. It has been six months since Max was fitted with his LVAD, and he is sick enough to die at any time. At 12:21 a.m., exactly twenty minutes after the offer is made, the Freeman returns the hub's call. The answer is a resounding yes. A heart this young, this healthy, and this beautifully preserved cannot possibly be turned down. It seems scarcely conceivable that two and a half days ago, this same heart—this living lifeline for Max—was inert and unbeating, in a state of cardiac arrest, for over forty minutes. For all that time, the only blood that flowed through its coronary arteries was via the roadside CPR, that a junior doctor, not one full year into his medical practice, scrambled to teach members of the public to deliver. Through nothing more technical than amateur, hopeful, desperate chest compressions—and the indefatigable impulse of a human heart to beat—Keira's organs received just enough oxygen to remain in a sufficient state of health to be gifted onward to others. The what-ifs are dizzying to contemplate. If Nick Hillier, the junior doctor on the scene, had been driving a car rather than riding a motorbike, and so was destined never to reach the scene of the crash. If he had chosen not to weave his way past the stationary cars, whether through fatigue, or distraction, or less stalwart resolve to check whether his newly minted medical skills could be of use to the casualties. If the paramedics had been unable to restart Keira's heart. If the shock of her blood loss had proved irreversible. So many ifs, such a far-fetched convergence. And yet, serendipitously, in the face of such steep odds, we are here in this moment of absolute altruism in which Keira's parceled parts, given by Joe and Loanna and their family without hesitation, are in the act of being assigned to others, to children and adults approaching death's door, whose lives they may genuinely save. In a tempestuous, fragile world, it is enough to make a person believe in miracles.

Throughout the night, the rest of Keira's organs are offered. At 3:30 a.m., one hospital accepts her liver. Shortly afterward, another hospital accepts the first kidney. Keira's organs are being allocated to others, even while her heart still beats. It is both the last thing in the world a parent wants to happen, and everything Joe hopes she can bequeath to others. Three hundred miles away from the hub in Bristol, Ward 23 at the Freeman is alive with purpose. There are parents to notify, operating theaters to book, surgeons to put on standby, the emaciated boy with white-blond hair to prepare—all the logistics that must proceed perfectly, seamlessly, because the slightest hiccup could end up costing Max what may be his last chance of a future.

Back in Bristol, with all of Keira's organs now accepted, the co-ordinator contacts the NHS National Organ Retrieval Service. Like the hub, NORS teams operate around the clock, 365 days a year, to retrieve organs from deceased donors as quickly as possible. A single team comprises a minimum of five people: a lead surgeon, an assistant surgeon, a transplant practitioner, a scrub nurse, and a donor care physiologist. Each team is typically on call for NORS for twenty-four hours at a stretch, in addition to their ordinary day jobs. There are sixteen such teams in the UK, of which ten are abdominal and six are cardiothoracic. The latter, responsible for retrieving hearts and lungs, are based in Birmingham, Glasgow, London, Manchester, Cambridge, and Newcastle.[1] That night, the first on-call cardiothoracic team is the one in Cambridge. The transplant coordinator in the city's Royal Papworth Hospital receives a call from the hub informing them that a pediatric heart needs retrieving first thing in the morning. Retrievals are typically rushed, middle-of-the-night affairs—time is of the essence—but in this case, the delay is in order to respect Keira's family's need to say goodbye to her without feeling pressured. Despite the precarious clinical state of so many patients awaiting organs, the transplant service always—and rightly—makes treating the donor family with humanity and kindness their first concern. Keira is emphatically not a warehouse of spare parts, she is a little girl, adored and cherished, who will be treated as such until the very end.

———————

At 5 a.m., Pradeep Kaul's eyes snap open. His fingers search reflexively for his phone while his conscious brain takes a moment to come round. "You know, we are human beings at the end of the day, we are not superhuman. For a second you think about sleep, but the moment you wake up properly, then you are on a mission, all you care about is the job you need to do. In the transplant continuing care unit I see how the recipients' lives are changed forever, how they can lead such fruitful lives after this. It's one of the things that keeps us going, for sure."

Pradeep, a consultant in cardiothoracic surgery at the Royal Papworth Hospital, is the lead retrieval surgeon on call that night. He and the other members of his team must arrive at the Royal Papworth within the hour. Their job, when they get to Bristol, is to retrieve Keira's heart in such a way that it incurs minimal damage during surgery. After that, the heart will be delivered into another team's hands—the surgeons waiting at the Freeman Hospital to transplant it into Max. As Pradeep drives through Cambridgeshire in the soft dawn light, he considers what the coordinator has just told him: that the person whose heart he will be retrieving is a nine-year-old child. "I've been doing this for a very long time, but I still feel like I conduct myself a little differently with children. We get more emotionally drained on pediatric retrievals than we would on adult retrievals. You become more pensive, reflecting on life, and you think more about the donor than you would otherwise. What happened to them? How did it come to this?"

Pradeep, who speaks twice as quickly and with twice as much energy as the average person, sports unruly black eyebrows and a luxuriant mustache. Born in Srinagar, Kashmir, in India, even as a child he would boil his father's scissors to ensure they were sterile before attacking with gusto his brothers' splinters, scrapes, and other minor injuries. Surgery was in his blood. It was during his surgical training in England that he became hooked on transplant. "It's the one sort of surgery where we really practice medicine as well. It involves immunology, critical care, immune suppression, all the other bits which mean it's not just stitching and walking away. The best thing is seeing how it changes people. I remember one patient, a tall guy who'd been diagnosed with dilated cardiomyopathy. When he came to us, he couldn't breathe, he couldn't walk—he was dying. Then, when we transplanted him, he was suddenly doing laps on the ward. So you have instant gratitude in transplant; you can see the outcome straightaway."

Also on her way to the Royal Papworth is transplant practitioner Clair Ellis, a highly experienced former transplant nurse whose role is of vital importance. Clair's responsibility is organ preservation and perfusion. She must ensure the heart is ideally "perfused"— or receives optimal blood flow—at all times so that its chances of being damaged due to lack of oxygen are minimized. "When the time comes to remove a heart, we run a solution through it called St. Thomas's cardioplegia. Part of my job is to calculate the correct amount of cardioplegia needed for the weight of the donor, and to gather together the right number of bags and iceboxes and lines and all the other equipment that's necessary. The scrub nurse does the same for the surgical instruments, all of which have to be sterile. Everything is logged, the timings, the quantities, because you cannot make a mistake; the timings are critical."

A van much like an ambulance is loaded with the seven-member team and all the equipment, before its driver sets off on the three-hour journey to Bristol. It is just after 7 a.m. "Sometimes fatigue takes over and you sleep for a bit, even if you didn't want to," says Pradeep. "But what we tend to do is discuss the case. We rely on each other's expertise. These retrievals can be very long and drawn out. They run at their own pace and we can't expedite that. So you have to think, 'Okay, it's going to happen in its own way.' You need to be quite zen and make sure nobody gets edgy about delays, even though you all know delays matter."

————

Specialist nurse in organ donation Sarah Crosby is on her way into Bristol, full of trepidation. "I'd only been in the job for a year and this was my first solo pediatric case. I was very anxious. I think it was the fear that the family's grief was going to be overwhelming and I wouldn't know how to manage it. I was putting my own fears onto the case, expecting people to be on the floor, crying and wailing." Before she went to bed, Sarah made sure she knew every detail of the case backward—Keira's injuries, her family situation, anything that might help her prepare for whatever she was going into. Despite her nerves and fitful sleep, she makes a point of arriving early the next morning to provide relief for her colleague, who has been there overnight.

For a SNOD, the day of a retrieval is a role of two extremes. On the one hand, you are there to give the donor family all the attention, support, and compassion they need. Catastrophic loss has invariably stunned them at exactly the time when events could not be more bewildering or overwhelming. You are a guide, a grief counselor, an interpreter, a psychotherapist. At the same time, you are responsible for coordinating all the logistics from the donor end that will culminate—hopefully—in a successful transplant. The recipient's life rests in your hands every bit as much as those of the transplant surgeons. Emotions simply cannot get the better of you. All this weighs heavily on Sarah's mind as she drives toward Bristol. She notices the sky: empty, flawless, the start of an idyllic summer's day. As she walks toward the PICU, Joe Ball happens to be taking a short break with Keely and Katelyn, perhaps in the cafeteria for breakfast. Sarah arrives outside Keira's cubicle. She knocks, hesitates, takes a deep breath and enters.

"I can still picture the room so vividly," says Sarah. "Her bed was directly in front of you as you walked in. I remember seeing the most beautiful nine-year-old girl asleep on a bed. She was perfect, you couldn't see anything wrong. It is always such a hard, hard image to see. Her sisters had plaited her hair and her nails were this gorgeous orange. She looked just like she'd been at a sleepover with her siblings. It was so peaceful. And then Dad walks in, full of energy, full of pride. He went straight over and kissed his daughter and made a fuss of her, and her sisters just snuggled in with her. I was in absolute awe of Joe. I can't imagine the pain he was feeling, this incredible man who had always been so loving, but his head was held high—he did it for his daughters. I just can't imagine the strength it would have taken for him to have walked into the room like that."

As Sarah introduces herself, she is struck by the family's enormous sense of pride in what Keira is going to do for others. "As far as Katelyn and Keely were concerned, it wasn't a secret, it was something to shout from the rooftops. They were so, so proud of her becoming a donor. It gave this loss a meaning. It was something so tragic and the only way they could fathom it was through the fact that she was meant to go on and save people's lives." Sarah carefully explains what will happen next. A surgical team is on its way and will arrive around mid-morning. Then it will be time for the family to say goodbye to her. Sarah will accompany Keira into the operating theater, where she will be given an anesthetic, just like any other patient. After the surgeons retrieve her organs, she will be returned to her room in the PICU, ready to be reunited with her family. Joe, Katelyn, and Keely give the impression of taking it all in stride, continuing to lavish affection on Keira. "I had always expected pediatric death to feel really somber, and of course it is," says Sarah. "But this room wasn't somber. There was no tiptoeing around this poorly child. This room was about love. This room was about hope and pride and two sisters who adored their baby sister, and grandparents and aunties and uncles, and music playing, and love. There was so much love in that room, it was beautiful. I think that's what really shocked me."

———

Jemma Evans, the nurse who has cared so attentively for Keira for the last two days, was meant to have Wednesday off, but has asked if instead she could work today's shift. She feels a need to see it through, to support Keira and her family, whom she has come to know so well, until the very end. "Keira was the first child I cared for throughout the whole organ donation journey. People say, 'Gosh, it must be so hard looking after a child in intensive care, how do you do your job?' And it *is* hard, but they aren't our children. It's almost as though, because the parents are there, you can behave in a very loving, very caring way towards the child, but you're slightly holding yourself back inside. It doesn't feel the same as it would if it was your child. The fact that Joe, Katelyn, Keely, and the extended family were there showing so much love with their presence and their words and their touch allowed us, as professionals, to get on with the technical side of the job."

Now that a theater is on standby and a retrieval team en route, the nurses try to stay out of the way as much as possible, giving Keira's family the space and privacy they need. The most pressing issue is enabling Loanna to spend some time with her daughter. Logistically, this is no small matter. A nurse, doctor, and hospital porter accompany her in a wheelchair from the adult ICU to the PICU. Her injured leg is outstretched in front of her, having been pinned and plated two days earlier by the trauma team. She just manages to hold her daughter's hand. Physically, Loanna is clearly in enormous pain, but what strikes Sarah Crosby more than anything is her emotional anguish. "She was like a shell. She couldn't speak a word. I don't think she had the energy to cry. She looked like everything had been taken from her. All I wanted to do as a nurse was to go and hold her, put my arms around her. She knew it was the last time she was ever going to see her daughter. She was absolutely broken. What she needed was her daughter to sit up in bed and say, 'Mum, it's okay—I'm going to be okay,' but none of us could give her that. She was destroyed."

Far away in Newcastle, a transplant coordinator in the Freeman Hospital is in constant contact with Sarah Crosby. Alison Davidson has been a nurse at the Freeman for over fifteen years, the last eleven of which have been in her current role. Today, her job is the mirror image of Sarah's. Alongside supporting Max and his family, she will manage every last detail of his transplant's logistics. Unless the surgical team in Bristol perfectly coordinates their retrieval with the surgeons who will be simultaneously dissecting out Max's heart in Newcastle, there is a very real possibility that the heart could be unusable. Alison's role is to ensure that does not happen. Like everyone, she knows that a heart should remain on ice for no more than four hours, otherwise the lack of oxygen may cause irreversible damage. Alison's mantra, which she repeats obsessively to Sarah in every phone call, is to remember the LVAD. Whatever happens, do not forget the LVAD. What she means by this is that the length of time it will take the team in Newcastle to surgically extract Max's heart is unknown because the LVAD will be deeply embedded in scar tissue, requiring painstaking and meticulous dissection. Under no circumstances, therefore, should the surgeons in Bristol proceed to cross-clamp Keira's aorta—thus terminating the blood supply to her heart—before Alison has given the all clear.

Throughout the morning, Sarah and Alison have been speaking to each other every fifteen or twenty minutes to coordinate activities, but now it is time for Sarah to focus solely on Keira. Final hours are ebbing into final minutes. Soon, Keira's last moments with her family will be upon them, and no one in the room is unaware of this. As soon as Loanna is taken back to adult intensive care, Katelyn and Keely cuddle up to their sister, talking and singing to her, laughing, patting her, adding another coat of polish to her resplendent nails. "I wish the girls knew how incredible that was to watch," says Sarah, "because they were so, so brave. It's not like they didn't know. Of course they knew their sister was going to die. Of course they did. They just wanted to give her this final love. They were so strong to be able to do that." Joe is adamant that when Keira returns from her surgery, she would want to be wearing a party dress. "He suddenly said, 'I'm going to go shopping in Bristol to find her a pink party dress.' He wanted her to have the most beautiful classic princess dress," says Sarah. Shortly before 11:30 a.m., the Royal Papworth retrieval team arrives at the hospital. While Sarah heads off to brief them, Joe rushes to a nearby department store to find something magical for his youngest daughter to wear.

Inside the handover room, there are at least twenty people—two whole retrieval teams, abdominal and cardiothoracic, plus assorted theater staff from Bristol. Shortly, they will all be squeezed into the operating theater. Everyone is tense, raring to go. It is, to say the least, a daunting audience. Sarah must suppress any shred of emotion she is feeling in order to lead the handover with clipped efficiency. "It's about putting on a different hat. We can't give all that emotion to the surgeons. That's not good in any sense. They have got such an incredible job to do in the next six, seven, eight hours. They can't be dealing with that level of emotion. So you don't share it with anybody apart from your nursing colleagues on PICU. You take a lot of that emotion and keep it inside yourself, locked away." She begins. It takes over half an hour of bullet-point logic to plot the details of Keira's case. Her clinical state, the extent of her injuries, the plan for each organ, her body map findings, her past medical and surgical history.

Finally, Sarah has answered every question the surgical teams have. As always, she finds herself deeply moved by their attention to detail and desire to get it right. "With any pediatric organ donation, everyone wants the absolute best for the recipients. Everyone is going the extra mile. This is not just the life of our child in our PICU, this is potentially six other children's lives. I think you see the absolute best in the NHS at that point. It's everyone pulling out all the stops to make sure we only go to theater when the family is ready. If Dad needs a couple of extra minutes, then that's what happens. If he needs to say goodbye at the theater doors, that's what happens. There is no textbook for how you lose a child. So whatever that family needs to get through the next twenty-four hours, we pride ourselves on going above and beyond to achieve that."

Leaving the surgical teams to make their final preparations in theater, Sarah returns to Keira's room to find that Joe has just returned from his emergency shopping trip. A brand-new party dress, all sparkles and taffeta, is suspended from a hanger to the side of Keira's bed. "The girls had put it up there. It was just hanging up waiting for her, like she was going to a party." When Sarah tells the family that the retrieval team is ready, the mood in the room shifts, darkens. "The atmosphere changed. It was like we had reached the end of the road and the only next step was for her to go and have her operation. All I can remember is Joe. There were others there, too, but I only remember Joe. He didn't want to walk to the theater doors; he wanted to say goodbye to Keira in the room. I think he was hanging on by a thread. It was almost like he had given all his strength in the last few hours to get to where he was. The fact that we were taking Keira away now signified that he was losing his youngest baby girl. But I didn't see him cry in front of Keira. I don't even think I saw him cry in front of the two girls. He was on dad duty mode the whole time. He was composed and strong and proud, setting an incredible example to the girls. He talked to Keira for a long time. Then he just kissed her on the forehead and said something like 'I know you are going to go and do something incredible now.' But you could tell he would have done anything to have stayed in that room with her for just a little bit longer."

At 12:30 p.m. the theater team arrives on the PICU. Jemma intercepts them outside Keira's room and asks them to wait while she checks on the family. "It usually takes a few minutes for a family to say their final goodbyes and then the theater team come in, disconnect the ventilator, put on the hand ventilation circuit, and escort the child to theater," says Jemma. Together with Sarah, a PICU consultant, and the theater team, Jemma accompanies Keira, still wearing her Mickey Mouse pajamas, out of the PICU and toward the operating theater. "It was the smoothest transfer you could imagine," Sarah recalls. "Everybody would have known about the case, even if they didn't know who Keira was. So all the doors were being opened for us. Everyone was trying to do their little bit to help. But then, of course, came the moment when the theater doors had swung closed behind us. We were in the theater. This was it."

Judgment

In 2015, the *Bulletin of the Royal College of Surgeons of England* caused something of a stir when it published the provocatively titled paper "A Stressful Job: Are Surgeons Psychopaths? And If So, Is That Such a Bad Thing?"[1] The two authors, both of whom were trauma and orthopedic surgeons, speculated that since doctors experienced significant stressors in their careers like excessive working hours, night shifts, and medical lawsuits, it would not be surprising if some of the traits known to be associated with a psychopathic personality—such as a preternatural calmness under pressure, or an apparent indifference to human suffering when making life-or-death decisions—were selected out in those who rose to the top of the medical profession.[2] In order to test their hypothesis that psychopaths were overrepresented among the ranks of hospital consultants versus the general population, they assessed the personality traits of 172 doctors using the official Psychopathic Personality Inventory.[3] Controversially, they found doctors did indeed appear to have higher-than-average psychopathy scores, with one of the criteria—"stress immunity"—being particularly prevalent among surgeons. The authors concluded that psychopathic traits might, perversely, lead to better patient care since too much empathy could cause doctors to turn away from their patients, finding it too painful to emotionally engage with them.

The acclaimed British heart surgeon Stephen Westaby, now retired, not only agrees with the assessment that he is a psychopath, but positively celebrates it. He attributes his surgical success to a radical personality change caused by a head injury sustained in his youth:

> At medical school I went from being a nice, considerate young man who wouldn't say boo to a goose to an aggressive young man who by then was fit to be a heart surgeon. I got injured playing rugby—a bi-frontal head trauma that causes psychopathy—and I had a complete personality change. If you look at psychopaths' brains on MRI scans, they're short of grey matter at the front. I wasn't born like that, but somebody provided me with it.[4]

In his autobiography, *Fragile Lives*, it is with evident pride that Westaby self-identifies as having character traits that set him apart from ordinary people: "We were not normal people. Most rational young men would be paralysed by fear at the thought of carving open someone's chest, then stopping, opening and repairing their heart. But I did this day after day. We were fuelled by testosterone, driven by adrenalin."[5]

This idea of open-heart surgeons as psychopathic outliers is, perhaps, the logical extension of the reverence and wonder in which they were held in the 1960s, these fearless, larger-than-life mavericks who cut, thrust, cleaved, and conquered where the rest of us were too timid to tread. They boldly went, they played gods with hearts, they were clearly semi-deities themselves. Christiaan Barnard did nothing to dispel this impression. Decades after carrying out the first-ever heart transplant, Barnard told fellow heart surgeon David Cooper, "You know, I've stood at patients' beds when they died and . . . I feel so upset, but I realize what I'm really upset about is that, when I write up my series of operations, I have one more mortality. It wasn't really the death of the patient—it is the ego that is hurt. I should not have had a death with this particular type of operation; I'm too good for that."[6]

Such honesty is disconcerting. Barnard appears to be saying that when he witnessed one of his patients die, he was distressed not primarily because someone for whose life he had been responsible was dead, but because the death was detrimental to his surgical results and, more fundamentally, was an affront to his ego. The psychopathic feature of coldheartedness, defined in the Psychopathic Personality Inventory as "guiltless, callous, unreactive to others' distress," seems applicable.[7] Yet Barnard was also renowned for being devoted to his patients' post-operative care, sometimes spending hours, even days, at their bedside to ensure they had the best possible outcome.[8] Not obviously the behavior of a psychopath. Perhaps the only clear conclusion is that psychopathy, like humanity, is complicated, and glib assertions are best avoided.

What is indisputable is Barnard's exceptional drive. In 1955, he moved from South Africa to America to train with the renowned group of heart surgeons in Minnesota, where he worked night and day to squeeze a six-year training program into two years.[9] On his return, he set up South Africa's first open-heart surgery program at Groote Schuur Hospital, Cape Town, and an experimental laboratory in which to practice transplants on dogs. By 1967, however, the front-runner in the race to transplant a human heart was, as mentioned earlier, Stanford's Norman Shumway, with his remarkable track record of over three hundred canine heart transplants. Such was Shumway's skill in managing immunosuppression that some of the dogs were still alive over a year after their transplant without succumbing to either infection or rejection. Barnard, by contrast, had transplanted only forty-eight hearts in dogs, of which the longest survivor had died after ten days.[10] Barnard later commented to David Cooper, "We perfected the surgical technique in the laboratory. We never tried to get long-term survival. All we were interested in was perfecting the surgical technique." The technique Barnard adopted in 1967 was directly copied from Shumway and his colleague Richard Lower, leading to charges from medical contemporaries that he piggybacked on the skills of others in order to steal their thunder: "Barnard's preparatory experimental work in heart transplantation was negligible, and many Americans to this day think he jumped the gun to get ahead of the front runners in the field."[11]

There were three obstacles to transplanting a human heart in the 1960s, of which surgical technique was the most easily overcome. The other two—how to manage rejection of the heart in the recipient and how to obtain a healthy donor heart in the first place, given that brain death had yet to be recognized medicolegally—were more daunting. When Barnard tried to persuade the head of cardiology at Groote Schuur, Val Schrire, to permit him to attempt a transplant in one of his patients, Schrire's response was blunt: "Your dogs don't live very long. You should get longer survivors before you try this."[12] However, in his own words, Barnard "plagued Val Schrire day and night" for a patient until, finally, he relented.

When Barnard first scrutinized a coronary angiogram of Louis Washkansky's heart, he was astonished to view an organ so wrecked it was "beyond the reach" of medicine or surgery. "I have never seen such massive destruction—are you sure this man's still alive?" he asked Schrire.[13] Washkansky, fifty-five, a former amateur boxer, had suffered three previous heart attacks. In addition to his end-stage heart failure, he had diabetes, liver failure, kidney failure, and active cellulitis—a skin infection on his left calf. His quality of life was wretched. Too breathless to leave his hospital bed and grossly swollen with retained fluid, he was, in effect, waiting to die. When Barnard offered him the chance of a potential cure in the form of a heart transplant, he accepted without hesitation, having nothing—or so it seemed—to lose. In a conversation with Washkansky's wife, Ann, Barnard put Louis's chances of survival at 80 percent, despite his having multiple comorbidities including the leg infection that had not responded to treatment. A virulent strain of the bacterium klebsiella had been cultured from his calf. With Washkansky on immunosuppressants to prevent rejection, the organism could be lethal. When intravenous antibiotics failed to clear the infection, Barnard therefore tried irradiating Washkansky's leg with cobalt—without success. Nevertheless, he had his recipient. Now he just needed a donor.

Although the French doctors Pierre Mollaret and Maurice Goulon had coined the phrase *coma dépassé* in 1959—the term that swiftly became synonymous with brain death—there was no agreed upon clinical or medicolegal definition of brain death anywhere in the world in 1967.[14] Mechanical ventilation had created the tantalizing possibility for transplant surgeons of a supply of perfectly preserved donor organs retrieved from the living bodies of patients with dead brains, but the concept remained ethically fraught. One of Norman Shumway's concerns about attempting the first human heart transplant, for example, was whether the public was fully prepared for the notion that a person could be dead while their heart was still beating.[15] Fortuitously for Barnard, in South Africa at the time the legal definition of death was comparatively lax. So long as two doctors agreed that a person was dead, then legally speaking they were.[16]

On December 2, 1967, a young woman and her mother were crossing a busy street in Cape Town to buy cake for afternoon tea when a driver veered across their path. In the collision that followed, Myrtle Darvall was killed instantly, while her twenty-five-year-old daughter, Denise, sustained catastrophic head injuries. Denise, nicknamed Denny by her family, was a fan of opera, Joan Sutherland, and Barbara

Cartland novels.[17] She was rushed by ambulance to Groote Schuur Hospital and placed on a ventilator, with two severe skull fractures and no detectable brain activity. By nine o'clock that evening, all efforts at resuscitation were abandoned. Denise's father gave permission for her organs to be transplanted and Barnard was notified of a potential donor. On learning that her blood group was compatible with Washkansky's, he immediately rushed to the hospital.

As soon as Barnard arrived, the senior neurosurgeon of Groote Schuur Hospital, Dr. Peter Rose-Innes, confirmed that, in his view, Denise Darvall was brain dead. Barnard regarded it as a given that brain death was synonymous with "legal death" or "total death," as he put it. In an extraordinary passage in his autobiography, he stated that Jesus Christ himself would certainly have been an organ donor: "Christ on the Cross would have done it, too. If there had been a possibility of doing a transplant, of using one of his organs, he would have given it immediately. He had given his whole life for mankind. So he would have given part of it for part of mankind."[18] As far as Barnard was concerned, Darvall was now a "biological vegetable" and the retrieval of her heart could proceed immediately.

The operation began at 1 a.m., Barnard leading a team of thirty surgeons, anesthesiologists, nurses, and technicians, including his brother, Marius. Once he had opened Washkansky's chest and connected him to the heart-lung machine, he asked for Darvall's ventilator to be switched off. Everyone in theater waited for her heart to stop beating. Five minutes passed, then ten, then fifteen. Remarkably, despite its lack of oxygen, the young, healthy heart continued indefatigably. Barnard was painfully aware that the more time elapsed, the greater the chances of the heart being irreparably damaged by ischemia. In his account of the surgery, he insists that he nevertheless kept waiting for Darvall's ECG to become a perfect flatline—and for a further three minutes after that—before instructing a colleague to cut out the heart. For the next thirty years, he maintained in public that he had wanted to be categorically certain that the heart had stopped beating of its own accord before opening her chest. However, after Barnard's death in 2001, Marius gave an interview to the journalist Donald McRae in which he stated that this was untrue. In fact, said Marius, while they were waiting in theater, he had asked Christiaan if he could inject Darvall with densely concentrated potassium in order to hasten a cardiac arrest. Christiaan had "nodded his assent" at Marius, who duly administered the potassium.[19] Thus the moment of cessation of Darvall's heartbeat was brought about by the Barnard brothers themselves.

Thereafter, the technical process of transplanting the new heart was surprisingly straightforward. Through his years of practicing on the hearts of dogs, Barnard had mastered the techniques required to seamlessly connect artery to artery, vein to vein with flair and confidence. Shortly after dawn—and after several shocks from a defibrillator—the team watched in awe as Denise Darvall's heart, newly sutured into place, resumed its beat inside the butterflied chest of Louis Washkansky.

––––––––

During the years they spend learning their craft, every surgeon-in-training will at some stage be taught the same surgical aphorism. A good surgeon is one who knows *how* to operate. A better surgeon is one who knows *when* to operate. But the best surgeon of all is one who knows when *not* to operate. On Ward 23 in the Freeman Hospital, no one had more expertise in transplant than consultant cardiothoracic surgeon Asif Hasan. A consummate communicator, he never directly revealed his concerns at Max's bedside, but he was worried. As late spring turned to summer, Max's dad, Paul, began to notice that each time Asif visited Max on his morning ward round, his gaze was more intent, more piercing. "Mr.

Hasan was very enigmatic, very calm. He would stand with his arms folded looking at Max, assessing him. He would be standing a little way from us, staring at Max. You could tell he was thinking, Is he going to be well enough for a transplant? Or would they have to take him off the list, easing him into the end of his life?"

In 1994, when Asif became a consultant surgeon, his workload was astounding. On average, he would perform around four hundred open-heart surgeries a year. Several times a week, after finishing in theater, he would remain with his patient throughout the night. "If I did anything complex, I wouldn't go home. I would sleep on the intensive care unit because there wouldn't be anybody else with experience on the unit overnight. I needed to be there. In the end, I said to my CEO, 'Look, my life is hell. I'm sleeping two or three nights a week in intensive care. You have got to get ICU doctors in at night.'" During one particularly grueling eighteen-month period, Asif was the only consultant heart surgeon in his hospital. "I was completely on my own, working a one-in-one on-call. That meant you were permanently on call—for eighteen months. No holidays, no days off, no nothing. That kind of pressure can really break you. That is the reality of this kind of job."

Today, Asif is close to retirement, having been a transplant surgeon for over thirty years. In total, he has transplanted more than five hundred hearts or hearts and lungs combined. Growing up in Karachi in Pakistan, he knew with absolute certainty from the age of ten what he wanted to do with his life. "I didn't want to be a doctor, I wanted to be a surgeon. It had to be surgery. I suppose there was a bit of romance in it. I was eleven when the first heart transplant occurred, and I remember it clearly. Christiaan Barnard was a hero. It was a huge event, and we were excited, and it was talked about a lot." A gentle and quietly spoken man, Asif has a hawklike intensity. Colleagues and families find themselves drawing in closer, not wanting to miss a word he says. Brooding, watchful, it is hard to imagine him ever resting or sleeping.

Over the years, the toll of cardiothoracic surgery on Asif's family has been immense. "The family takes a big hit, you know? The big surgeries always seem to happen during the night. You never see your children—you're that sort of guy. When you're in theater, you have to park the fact that the one thing you told your wife before you left for work was 'I will definitely be back for dinner,' and now, of course, you won't be there. Or, your daughter has told you she needs to go to a Christmas party, and now, you know, you're not going to be able to take her. All that sort of stuff is going on in the background." If there is a reason his family—he is married with one daughter—has remained intact and loving, it is, he says, down to his immensely understanding and saintly wife. But also, crucially, when he does leave the hospital, he never, ever discusses his work at home. "I could just be a greengrocer or something like that. I remember, years ago, coming back completely exhausted during that period of continual work. I just lay down on the sofa—I'd been up all night transplanting—and said to my four-year-old daughter, 'Please can I have a glass of water?' And she looked at me and said, 'Oh, Daddy, you are just so lazy. You should get it yourself.' I think that completely puts you in your place in a wonderful way. It's important."

What exercised Asif in early summer 2017 was the precariousness of Max's situation. He knew that too often in transplant surgery, the aphorisms do not apply. The tragedy of the transplant waiting list is that it dictates the timings of a surgery more often than any doctor can. In Max's case, there was simply no choice in the matter. The instant a suitable heart became available, Asif would have whisked him into theater. But the scarcity of pediatric donor organs meant no such heart could be found. Although Max's left ventricle remained relatively well supported by the LVAD, the right side of his heart was now failing with alarming rapidity, causing his liver and kidneys to fail, too. If he waited much longer, Max would cease to be fit enough for surgery and his management would shift from transplant to end-of-life care.

One day, the ward suggested that Emma and Paul receive a lesson in how to give CPR. Ostensibly, this was to enable them to take Max off the ward for short periods without a nurse escort. "They said, 'If you are going to take him off the ward by yourself, you have to have CPR training in case he has a cardiac arrest,'" says Paul. "I felt it was a bit of a hint. Deep down I thought the CPR training was because something could happen at any time and therefore we needed to be prepared." Then Emma and Paul heard about another boy in the heart unit, roughly Max's age and also waiting on the super-urgent transplant list, who had suddenly deteriorated and started screaming. The form of LVAD with which the boy was fitted, the Berlin Heart, had caused a massive stroke. To his mother's horror, he died in a matter of minutes. "I realized a lot of Max's destiny was going to be pot luck," says Emma. "It was pot luck who survived and who died. It made me feel like we were in some kind of macabre lottery where you would roll the dice one day and Max could have a good day, then you'd roll it the next day and that could be it. That's how it felt. Max was walking on a tightrope and at any moment he could just fall off."

Max's options were running out. The lowest point for Emma occurred when a doctor took her to one side in the ward playroom to tell her that the team was being forced to consider giving Max a Berlin Heart to support the right side of his heart, in addition to the LVAD he already had. "I just burst into tears. I was terrified. I said, 'If you do that, it's game over. If he has a Berlin Heart, I honestly don't think he will make it. I just don't think his body can cope with an LVAD and a Berlin Heart.'" Really, Emma was desperate to protect Max from the risk of a stroke caused by a Berlin Heart, having known the young boy on the ward who had died in precisely this manner. But in the absence of a donor heart, the reality of end-stage heart failure is that no option is a good option. Do nothing, and your patient dies. Use a mechanical device as a bridge to transplant, and your patient may die from a massive stroke. Use medications to help the heart to beat more forcefully, and you may cause their death from a fatal arrhythmia. Every course of action left open to the surgeons could save Max's life or kill him. It was as though Asif's king was being slowly checkmated by a twisted grand master with a heart of stone. Asif had to make the next move.

———

The life of Denise Darvall's heart inside the bony cradle of Louis Washkansky's chest spanned only eighteen days. Nevertheless, when the story broke that Christiaan Barnard had successfully performed the world's first heart transplant, it was heralded across the globe as a spectacular triumph of human endeavor, to rival Neil Armstrong and Buzz Aldrin's first moon landing two years later in 1969. One of Barnard's British contemporaries, Roy Calne, who would go on to perform Europe's first liver transplant and the world's first combined heart, liver, and lung transplant,[20] said of the media hype, "The first heart grafts were covered by the media on a scale equivalent to the news of a major war."[21] It was true. In a five-page cover story about the transplant entitled "The Ultimate Operation," *Time* magazine wrote that Barnard had "reached the surgical equivalent of Mount Everest."[22] The London *Sunday Times* reproduced on its front page the ECG generated by Darvall's heart inside Washkansky's chest, describing it as a "symbol of a medical miracle that has given hope to a man who had only days to live."[23] What no one understood at the time was that Washkansky still had only days to live.

At first, Washkansky appeared stable. He was given large doses of immunosuppressants and sealed inside a sterile plastic tent to try to protect him from bacterial infection. A few days after the surgery, he was well enough to smile, eat a little, and crack jokes with the nurses. By now, national and international journalists were besieging Groote Schuur Hospital, all clamoring for interviews. Washkansky, who had become the world's most famous patient, even managed to talk to a few of them. But by the fifth day he was sluggish, exhausted, and irritable. In his autobiography, Barnard describes Washkansky saying to him, "I've had enough. Leave me alone. . . . They're killing me. I can't sleep, I can't eat, I can't do anything. They're at me all the time with pins and needles, pins and needles."[24] His bloods had worsened, his kidneys were failing, and his heart rate had climbed to 150 beats per minute. Barnard, fearing rejection, drastically increased his immunosuppression in a frantic bid to reverse the decline. Meanwhile, the microbiology lab detected klebsiella in samples from Washkansky's mouth, rectum, and nostril. It was the same bacterium known to have been deeply entrenched in the infected wound on his leg prior to his surgery.

Barnard wrote that the transplant had given Washkansky "a remarkable state of well-being which lasted five days—five glorious days of new life for a man who had been dying. It was as though we had climbed out of the jungle onto an open plateau which extended without limit."[25] But was it? Washkansky was cocooned within a plastic bubble and recovering from his sternum being sawn in half and his ribs cranked apart, all while being subjected to potentially lethal doses of steroids. Over the next ten days he continued to deteriorate, with high temperatures, a rising white cell count, clinical evidence of bilateral pneumonia, and three different bacteria—klebsiella, pseudomonas, and pneumococcus—growing in his sputum. Barnard continued to ramp up the doses of immunosuppressants. By day fourteen, Washkansky was unable to stop himself urinating and defecating in bed and was in so much pain that he preferred to lie in his own diarrhea than "suffer the agony of movement." By day sixteen, he was blue from lack of oxygen. While still conscious—and despite his vocal protestations—an endotracheal tube was inserted down his nose and into his trachea in order to deliver more oxygen. The next day, Barnard weighed up whether to put him back on the heart-lung machine to buy him some time to recover from his pneumonia. At this point, Barnard's colleague Val Schrire drew the line, saying, "You'll increase his agony, and torment everyone else." A few hours later, Washkansky was dead.

Can Christiaan Barnard really be said to have acted in Louis Washkansky's best interests? Or had he allowed personal ambition and competitive zeal to override his clinical judgment? Did he operate for his patient's sake, or for his own? From a twenty-first-century perspective, the ethics of the first heart transplant are clearly questionable, not least regarding whether there was any genuinely informed consent to the procedure. But what really stands out to a contemporary physician are the abject misery and loss of dignity that characterized Washkansky's final days. The specialty of palliative medicine had scarcely been invented in the 1960s and the world's first purpose-built hospice, St. Christopher's Hospice in London, did not open until a few months before his transplant. The concept of a fate worse than death—for example, a death that is cruelly dragged out by futile treatments that cause a patient only pain and wretchedness—was rarely discussed by doctors in the 1960s.[26] In its place, medicine was dominated by paternalism, as exemplified by Barnard's conviction that he could speak for his patients, their families, the general public, and even on behalf of Jesus himself. Years later, in 1979, Barnard admitted in an interview in a Canadian medical journal that "I have a tremendous ego, I know that, and I must feed it, or I become miserable and unhappy. I have enjoyed world fame, beautiful women—and I have shunned none of it."[27]

Barnard unleashed a worldwide transplanting frenzy. In *Hearts Exposed: Transplants and the Media in 1960s Britain*, a cultural history of the UK's first heart transplants, historian Ayesha Nathoo describes how 1968 became "the year of the heart transplant," with over a hundred hearts transplanted in eighteen different countries, despite many of the surgical teams having negligible experience of managing rejection and immunosuppression.[28] Roy Calne believed that Barnard's love of the limelight made him partially responsible for the surgical scramble, commenting:

> Barnard toured the world as a "super-celebrity" and cardiac surgeons in other countries felt that they could also do this operation. They did not give sufficient consideration to the dangers of rejection and the lack of an effective regimen to handle it. Some surgeons were remarkably ignorant of the biology of transplantation. Nevertheless, it became a badge of machismo for each unit to announce its own heart transplant, preferably before the heart stopped beating.[29]

Statistically, Calne was vindicated. A paper published at the end of December 1968 showed that out of sixty-five patients to have received a new heart in the preceding twelve months, only half were still alive.[30] Another study demonstrated that two-thirds of the patients operated on in 1968 died within three months of their heart transplant.[31] In the face of the rising death toll, skepticism and hostility mounted in the media, too. When, for example, the *Guardian* reported news of the first UK heart transplant, performed in secrecy in May 1968, one consultant cardiologist quoted in the piece said that the surgery "almost amounted to cannibalism."[32]

The patient died of infection forty-six days later, and the surgeon, Donald Ross, only attempted two more heart transplants (both patients died in a matter of weeks) before choosing to abandon the procedure. He was unwilling to try again until the problem of rejection was resolved. The UK effectively introduced a moratorium on heart transplants for nearly a decade.[33] For some clinicians, what had once been seen as a medical miracle, met by the public with such hope and awe, had become synonymous with surgical hubris.

––––––––––

In 2019, the American author and *New Yorker* writer Malcolm Gladwell announced in a live public debate with fellow author David Epstein that he was going to offend all the medical doctors in the room. He wasn't exaggerating. "I honestly think that . . . the overwhelming majority of college graduates, given the opportunity, could be better-than-average cardiac surgeons," Gladwell said. "That is to say . . . if we put them through ten thousand hours of deliberate practice, they could all end up being good cardiac surgeons. I don't think there's any magical talent. In other words . . . if you're smart enough to get through college, you can be a great surgeon."[34]

The two authors were debating the secrets of success—specifically, what underpins truly exceptional greatness in sports, music, business, and anything else. Gladwell's recently published book *Outliers* had popularized the "10,000-hour rule," which suggests that no matter how much innate talent someone possesses, this level of practice is required before a high achiever can reach such an elevated pitch of performance that they may truly be described as an outlier.[35] During the debate, Gladwell projected onto medicine the idea that practice trumped talent, arguing that since surgery is a psychomotor skill, hard work was really all it took to become a halfway-decent surgeon. Any old graduate could do it. Gladwell plowed on. He actually had a very low opinion of the difficulty of cardiac surgery, he said, regarding operating on a person as not much harder than driving a car. "Driving is insanely complicated," he said, yet there is an "assumption that everyone can learn to drive in a safe way. We don't question that. There's no screening. My mother's eighty-three—she still drives." His conclusion? "If you can drive a car, you can ultimately cut into someone's heart."

Offended surgeons took to social media to push back against Gladwell's dismissal of their craft. What he had revealed above all, they pointed out, was his ignorance of what complex surgery actually entailed.[36] But the most interesting riposte to Gladwell—though it was not intended as such—came from Sir Barry Jackson, former serjeant surgeon to the queen and former president of the Royal College of Surgeons of England. In a speech in Oxford in 2018, Jackson addressed the specific topic: What makes an excellent surgeon?[37] His answers are brilliantly insightful for understanding the modern surgical mind. He points out that in the nineteenth century, in the absence of anesthesia, there was a simple, one-word answer to the question: speed. Robert Liston, for example, was revered for being able to whip off a leg in thirty seconds.[38] Then, around the turn of the twentieth century, boldness became the cardinal feature of great surgeons. But today, a plethora of different qualities is needed, and while manual dexterity and technical skill are clearly important, as per Gladwell, they are by no means sufficient for excellence. First-class judgment is at least as important, as demonstrated by a surgeon's ability to know when and when not to operate. So, too, are calmness under pressure, humility, team-working, self-awareness, a willingness to adapt and learn, good communication skills, high ethical standards, and the cardinal rule of doing to others as you would have done to yourself. Jackson adds: "The ability to communicate with patients and their relatives in a quietly confident way, at all times being honest and understandable, is part of the hallmark of a master surgeon. Arrogance or seeming superiority should be abhorred."[39]

When Asif Hasan was trying to weigh up the least worst option for his sickest patient, he had very little room for maneuver. But Emma's concerns about a Berlin Heart for Max were heard and, crucially, respected. There was one other option, an old-fashioned drug, little used in modern medicine. The team made it clear to Emma that if Max failed to respond to the drug, dobutamine, there was no real alternative to the Berlin Heart, but they were willing to try it first. Dobutamine would increase the contractility of the muscle of the heart, but it would also increase the risk of a fatal arrhythmia. It was a stopgap, not a long-term solution. Yet within twenty-four hours of starting the infusion, Max was noticeably brighter. "He'd perked up," says Emma. "I could see he was more alert. He started chatting to me. I think the decision to try dobutamine saved his life."

Retrieval

Theaters are a maze of gurneys and corridors, sharp corners and glaring lights, locked doors and peculiar smells. Nurses dart between rooms at such speed that their clogs squeak as they walk. Porters shift people like cargo, expediting deliveries of inert and anesthetized human forms on their way to recovery rooms that may or may not contain a window and natural light. Sometimes the playlist from a surgeon who likes her music loud wafts out from behind a set of closed swing doors. When rolling into this alien world of steel and sterility, masks and gowns, a child is granted the comfort of having a parent by their side. But not today. Joe is left in intensive care with a hole in his heart that collapses time. Keira has been moved alone through the hospital and light-years away from him. If she has already gone, as the doctors claim, then why does it feel as though she is being prized from his arms?

Inside the operating theater, some of the staff are struggling, too. You can see it on their faces, taut with the effort of clamping down their emotions. Many years ago, Christiaan Barnard sought to dismiss as "mythology and ritual" the reasons why other members of Denise Darvall's surgical team recoiled from "touching a beating heart in a body that had been declared clinically dead."[1] He implied that these sentiments were foolish and nonsensical. Yet the reframing of everything we thought we knew about death—its cold gray certainties, the pulse transfixed, the warmth erased—is not a formality. It upends everything our senses sing to us of life. And Barnard ignored the most obvious point of all. Across different cultures and eras, the desecration of dead bodies is a deep-seated taboo. Long past the moment when a person's heart has ceased to beat, past the point where flesh is cold, the human body, whether alive or dead, is not a resource to be plundered at will. Bone, sinew, flesh, hair—they make manifest the people whom we love and cherish. How could they be reducible, after death, to stuff and nothing more? Corteges and bouquets, processionals and laments, candles and incense, caskets and black ties, the ceremonies with which we honor the dead are acts not of logic but of love. An organ donor whose brain stem has died may be insensate, but humans are hardwired to treat each other with respect—and taking a scalpel to their soft warm flesh is no small matter at all.

It is for exactly this reason that, whenever possible, organ retrievals in the UK are preceded by a moment of honor, a practice shared by many countries around the world. NHS Blood and Transplant defines the moment of honor as "a respectful pause, taking place either before or after the retrieval operation. This moment brings together those who have cared for the donor, and is a time of reflection and appreciation of the selfless act of kindness and generosity from the donor and their family."[2] The moment is usually led by the specialist nurse in organ donation, and today is no exception. Inside the operating theater, a hush falls as Keira, escorted by an anesthesiologist, intensive care consultant, porter, and specialist nurse in organ donation Sarah Crosby, is wheeled in. Faces turn, eyes are riveted to the visage of a sleeping child. There are at least twenty people in this room, Sarah thinks, and yet, for a moment, it is as though every breath is collectively held. You could hear a pin drop. She begins to speak. "We are taking a moment now to give thanks to Keira and her family. Then we will be retrieving these incredible gifts to help save lives. We hope that these gifts will give life to other children, other recipients, and that they will do well from them and benefit from this absolute gift that Keira is giving. Please can we all now take a moment to think about Keira and how thankful we are to her and her family." Heads bow, eyes close, the air is thick with unvoiced thoughts. On the wall, the theater clock traces a full thirty seconds before anyone speaks again.

"I think for me what's overwhelming in that moment is the absolute privilege of being in the room," Sarah says. "The moment of honor is always very emotive, very moving, but it also gives everyone a chance to compose themselves. You're running on adrenaline because of how important the case is. You are hoping it is going to save lives. And this moment is also about trying to calm everyone, everyone's stress, because you want it to go as smoothly as possible. But mainly it is about honor. I feel lost for words trying to do it justice. For anyone who hasn't been involved in a moment of honor before, they say afterwards that they feel so grateful to have witnessed it and to have been able to give thanks to this incredible life-saving act that a person has given others."

Sometimes, holding the moment of honor prior to surgery feels too fraught for a surgeon, who is, after all, a human being, too. They cannot risk having their surgical poise clouded by emotion and ask for the moment to be postponed until after the retrieval has safely concluded. Today, though, both Pradeep Kaul, who will lead the cardiothoracic retrieval, and his counterpart responsible for the abdominal organs stand in silence while Sarah speaks. Pradeep's colleague from the Royal Papworth, transplant practitioner Clair Ellis, is also present. "These cases are an absolute tragedy, but at the same time, I'm thinking, 'I can't change it.' No one can, obviously," she says. "I know that we can save someone else, though—

you know, another child like Max who's been in hospital so long with parents who are just hoping one day he may get to go back to school. I think of that because it helps me. It's not about being selfish, it's just a way of justifying why we are there, doing what we're about to do. We have no control over anything except doing a good job. So once the material process starts, you become more disciplined, more focused, and you start worrying about the outcomes there and then, rather than what's left behind. Nobody tells you this when you start out doing transplant, but these are the ways you learn to cope." The moment of honor gives staff a chance to gather their emotions and send them packing, the better to do the job at hand. "From now on, I don't allow myself to think that there is a nine-year-old on the table, because I wouldn't be able to get my job done. I've detached myself and I'm focused on the process of helping these organs to save lives," says Sarah Crosby.

Aluminum gallium indium phosphide. The chemical components of the ceiling-mounted surgical lights sound less like a compound than an incantation. Their rays converge, pristine, piercing, on the diminutive human form below, the center of the room, and of the surgeons' universe. Someone sweeps a sterile drape into place, cleaving past from present, as much as head from body. It is a barricade designed to prevent the anesthesiologist breathing onto the opened chest and abdomen, potentially infecting them—but it also protects those wielding the scalpels from any unsteadying glimpse of humanity, above all the face of a child. The surgical field—for this is all that exists now, a rectangle demarcated by drapes of sea green— is bleached, bone-white, its contours burned away. Then the shock of the Betadine, daubs of coppery brown, the skin transmuted into sheets of rusted iron. No music in this theater, no playlists or chatter. The mood is somber as the teams arrange themselves in tiers around the table. Those closest to the center, the inner circle, are swathed like priests in sterile blue gowns, having scrubbed their hands and forearms raw with bubblegum-pink surgical soap. They reek of chlorhexidine gluconate. In his surgical headlamp, Pradeep looks like a miner readying himself to dig, to bring to the surface buried treasure. A heart, a liver, and two kidneys. You cannot put a price on four lives saved. A scrub nurse places a scalpel in an outstretched hand. Knife to skin. A ribbon of crimson. It is 1:50 p.m.

Fifteen minutes after the first incision, the thoracic and abdominal cavities are fully opened and Sarah has already sent photos of the liver to the recipient team. In a multi-organ retrieval, the cardiothoracic surgeons typically start last.[3] The reason for this is because the first phase of retrieval surgery involves dissecting away the tissues within which each organ is embedded. Because the heart is most susceptible to damage from being deprived of oxygen, it is left alone until the abdominal team has almost entirely untethered the liver and kidneys from the rest of the body.

The abdominal team begins by carefully dissecting away each kidney from the pouch in which it nestles, tucked just below the posterior ribs. The ligaments, attachments, and tissues must be freed, while keeping all things vascular intact—the renal arteries that keep pulsing warm red blood into each kidney, the renal veins that funnel the spent blood away. Next, the abdominal surgeons advance upward to the liver, where they repeat the same meticulous work, whittling and etching, until the organ is held in place only by the threads of the hepatic veins and arteries, poised to be excised in a moment.

Now, at last, it is Pradeep's turn. The pericardium gleams beneath the surgical lights. This is the tough fibrous sac protecting the beating heart within. Pradeep will split it with his scalpel's tip as surely as the skin of an overripe fig. He moves decisively, assertively, with confidence and grace. Suddenly—and it is as though thoracic waters break—the field is awash with pericardial fluid and there, unsheathed, is the heart itself, purple and red, pulsating, laboring, writhing, and gyrating with each contraction, this magnificent thing of force and beauty. It is impossible to tear your eyes from.

Pradeep coolly appraises the heart. It is measured and objectified: its size, shape, the contractile force of its ventricles, the rhythm of its beat, the pressures and flow of the blood through its four chambers. At 3:12 p.m. he delivers his verdict. It is a good heart, he confirms to Sarah. There is no evidence of damage.

Keira's organs can now be removed from her body. The order in which they are retrieved is determined by how long each of them can tolerate being deprived of oxygen. Studies show that excised hearts can endure cold ischemia—being embedded in ice to maintain a core temperature of approximately 4 degrees Celsius—for at most six hours when they come from young children.[4] Livers, on the other hand, can be cocooned in ice for up to twelve hours without survival rates being affected.[5] For kidneys, the most resilient organs of all, the ischemic time is up to twenty-four hours.[6] That means the order of retrieval is usually as follows: the heart is retrieved first, the lungs second, the liver third, and finally the kidneys.

It also means, incredibly, that in the US, kidneys and other organs are routinely transported on commercial airlines as though they were any other unaccompanied cargo. Prior to the 9/11 terrorist attacks, human organs traveling this way could at least be delivered straight to the pilots' cabin, where they often flew in the cockpit or under the immediate oversight of the flight crew. Changes put in place after 9/11, however, relegated unaccompanied donor organs to the cargo hold. Anyone who has ever had their luggage go missing or who has failed to make a connecting flight will recognize vividly the perils of treating a human organ as, essentially, baggage. A lost suitcase is an inconvenience; a misplaced organ puts someone's life on the line.[7] Between 2014 and 2019, for instance, nearly 170 organs were unable to be transplanted and almost 370 endured "near misses," with delays of two hours or more, due to transportation problems.[8] Once, for example, in 2018, Southwest Airlines flight 3606 from Seattle to Dallas was turned round in midair when the airline realized that a human heart—whose valves were intended for transplant into others—had been accidentally left behind in the hold.[9] "We've had organs that are left on airplanes, organs that arrive at an airport and then can't get taken off the aircraft in a timely fashion and spend an extra two or three or four hours waiting for somebody to get them," one transplant surgeon, David Axelrod from the University of Iowa, told NBC News.[10]

In the UK, the shorter distances across which donor organs are dispatched can often be spanned by covered road. If time is particularly tight, a light aircraft will be chartered. Today, there is no way Keira's heart can travel three hundred miles by road. Instead, it will be whisked from the operating theater straight into an ambulance, and from there to Bristol Airport, where a private plane will fly it to Newcastle, ready to be collected and rushed straight to the operating theater, where Max will be lying, draped and unconscious, his own chest splayed.

Sarah Crosby calls Alison Davidson in Newcastle to inform her that the Bristol team is almost ready to cross-clamp the aorta. But the response is not good. *Wait*, says Alison. *There's been a delay. We're still preparing to take Max to theater.* The Bristol team knows better than to press for further details. The choreography of transplants is always like this, intricate, unraveling, beholden to complications. They wait. At 4 p.m. Sarah calls Alison for an update and is told there will be at least another hour's delay. Max is now in theater, but the dissection of his LVAD is proving difficult and cannot be rushed. "You're waiting, waiting, waiting," says Sarah. "Literally everyone in the room just waiting to be told that, yes, you can cross-clamp, yes."

The theater in Bristol becomes increasingly hot and tense. Everything smells of chlorine and sweat. The annoyances that didn't exist in the heat of the moment—the itch of a label at the nape of the neck, a trickle of sweat approaching the coccyx—have come to the fore. Aching shoulders, sore feet, frustration at missing the kids' bedtime for the third night this week. Behind a drape, sequestered away from the rest of the team, the anesthesiologist obsessively checks and rechecks the infusions maintaining her patient's precarious limbo of warm pulsing lifelessness. The volatility of every vital sign—labile blood pressure, tachycardia, excessive urine output—are being stabilized with one aim in mind, the best possible perfusion of the organs.

It is not until 5:41 p.m. that Alison finally calls the team in Bristol to confirm they can go ahead and cross-clamp the aorta. Sarah has by now left the theater, many hours after the end of her shift. Joe, Katelyn, and Keely are still waiting in the PICU. Clair Ellis is on standby with the bags of icy-cold St. Thomas's cardioplegia solution she will flush through the heart to stop it beating. Pradeep gets to work. In moments, his hands are deep inside the chest. He inserts a cannula into the root of the aorta through which, in a moment, Clair will inject the cardioplegia solution. He wraps tourniquets around the superior and inferior vena cavae, ready to tighten them to stop the flow of blood into the heart. One final check before the point of no return. "Can we cross-clamp?" he asks the room. "Clamp," the specialist nurse in organ donation, Sarah's replacement, confirms. At 6:09 p.m., Pradeep places a clamp on the aorta and signals to the anesthesiologist to turn off the ventilator. The room grows quiet. The lungs deflate. All eyes on the still-beating heart. At 6:10 p.m., Clair opens the cardioplegia line and concentrated potassium begins to flow.

For nine years plus the months of Loanna's pregnancy—the 300 million beats of Keira's lifetime—this miniature machine has never faltered. The embryonic tissue of her heart began to pulse at a mere five weeks' gestation. The first of our organs to form, the last to die, it carried Keira safely through the earthquake of childbirth, it calmed and slowed in the cradle of Loanna's arms, it quickened with the joy of cuddling lambs on the farm, it exulted as Keira flew through the air on the back of her beloved pony, Charlie. Now translucent cardioplegia fluid floods the coronary arteries and takes only seconds to work. There is a quiver, a shiver, then the heart is still. Cold, instantaneous cardiac arrest, vital for preserving the astounding power that may yet save Max's life.

Everyone had known that Keira was already dead, but now the illusion of life is gone, too. No rise and fall of the chest, no flush of pink on soft cheeks. Swiftly, the body is purged of its blood, which Clair replaces with six bags of cardioplegia solution. The other organs cool rapidly. Inside the chest, Pradeep's fingers move like lightning. The fine dissection took place long ago. Now he works in arcs, in swaths, his single tool a pair of scissors. With impeccable strokes, he severs the superior and inferior vena cavae, then lifts up the heart in one hand to cut the four pulmonary veins that sit behind it. He lowers the heart back into the chest and severs the aorta and the pulmonary artery. The first time Pradeep did this, he was struck by the strangeness, but that was long ago. "You know, the whole space was filled up, but when we took the heart and the lungs out, the chest cavity was completely empty. Just empty. It was such an unfamiliar sight. But usually I find there is so much going on in our minds at this point, so many different people talking, a sort of melee, that it all happens very quickly and sometimes, by the time you're taking the heart out, you can't think of anything else because you're so focused on getting it right, just getting the organ out in the best possible condition."

Pradeep places the excised heart inside a clear plastic pouch filled with cardioplegia fluid. He places the pouch inside another, and then another, until, triple-bagged, the organ is laid on its bed of ice. Twelve minutes from the start of the cold perfusion, Keira's heart has been sealed inside a cooler filled to the brim with crushed ice. Two minutes after that, it has left the building. The hands of the abdominal surgeons, finally allowed to perform their own retrievals, are already buried in viscera.

———

What has passed through Joe's mind in the last six hours is impossible to imagine. He has decided, though, with predictable resolve, to honor his daughter all the way to the end, no matter how much it costs him. Outside the hospital, in a small ambulance bay some distance from the mayhem of the emergency department, four ambulances are lined up in a row, one for each organ. Joe stands a short distance away, a lonely figure, watching and waiting. When the crate containing Keira's heart is carried out to the first ambulance, he looks on in silence. *Autopsia*, from the ancient Greek, is the act of seeing for oneself. Joe's is not the autopsy of the forensic pathologist, who looks to learn, to unravel answers; this is something purer and deeper. "I had to see them load the boxes into ambulances and drive off with them. I had to see it," says Joe. He has chosen, simply, to bear witness. The porter passes the plastic container up into the hands of a paramedic. Though it is just the same as the coolers you might see on a beach or at a picnic, it contains nothing less than life itself. The doors close, the engine turns. As the ambulance moves out of the bay, toward the road, and round a corner, Joe's eyes do not leave it for a moment. For many long minutes after its departure, his gaze remains rooted to the spot where he has just observed his daughter's heart leaving him forever.

Back inside, the team from the Royal Papworth Hospital are the first to pack up, having completed the cardiac retrieval. As they prepare to leave the hospital, their driver arrives to forewarn them of Joe's presence outside. "He said to us, 'Just to let you know, the dad is outside,' to make sure we were prepared," says Clair Ellis. "We walked outside, and I remember seeing Joe standing some way away from the ambulances. I just felt for him so much. He wanted to see what an incredible thing Keira was doing, to see her gifts going off to help other people. I don't think I will ever forget that image of him standing there by himself with his arms folded."

Inside the operating theater, the liver and kidneys have been retrieved and are already on their way to other hospitals. The abdominal surgeons are now engaged in restoration work, the rebuilding of a hollowed body. Keira's family surrendered their beloved child and the very least the team can do in return is send her back to them with her dignity intact. The surgeons pack the hollows they created with surgical padding. They close the long incision that runs from the top of the sternum to the bottom of the abdomen with precise and elegant sutures. Everyone responsible for the prolongation of life—the surgeons, anesthesiologists, perfusionists, and transplant practitioners—now departs. Hope, in a sense, has left the room. In their wake, you look around and see only surgical detritus. The splashed and spilt blood, the discarded swabs, the dirtied instruments, the soiled cotton. It looks like something from a war zone. But what remains in those who have chosen to stay—in the nurses who will now perform Keira's last offices—is an abundance of invisible kindness.

Jemma Evans is one of them. "It was about closure. The job's not done until she's back with her family." Many of the theater nurses feel likewise. "We all knew that Joe was waiting," says Jemma. "We knew that Keira had been in theater for a really long time. Joe wanted to have her back, and having that many people to help meant we were able to do it much more quickly. All of these extra hands, helping and caring. I remember one of the theater nurses just sitting by her, by Keira's head, washing her hair, combing it beautifully, leaving it on the pillow to dry."

Beneath the searing theater lights, the nursing team washes every inch of Keira. Gentle hands, loving hands, restoring not health but humanity. Together they remove the lines and wires, placing clean white dressings over any visible punctures or incisions. Tenderly, they rub her hands and feet with lotion that smells of flowers. Keira is as cold and pale as marble. She could not be more clearly dead— and the point of the last offices is not to pretend otherwise. What these nurses are returning transcends appearance. This is a change of state, a restoration from surgical donor back to cherished human being. As they ease Keira's limbs into vivid pink taffeta—the party dress chosen by Joe, and which a porter has delivered from PICU to the theater—they know precisely what these rituals signify. You are loved. You mattered then, and you matter now, and you will matter always, forever. "Afterwards, I spoke to some of the theater staff," says Jemma. "They told me they'd found it really difficult to help with last offices, because it wasn't something that they normally do. But a lot of them said they were incredibly glad to have helped. They felt what was often missing for them when a child had died in theater was not being able to care for the child all the way through. They knew how much it would mean to the family. It was therapeutic to be involved."

It is late evening. Finally, Jemma is able to bring Joe, Katelyn, and Keely back to Keira's room on the PICU. The nurses have made a beautiful job of it. The lighting inside is soft and gentle, with electric candles dotting the tables and fairy lights strung from the ceiling. No more alarms or monitors, no needles or wires. Keira lies with closed eyes in a cloud of pink taffeta, her long golden hair spilling like honey over the edges of her pillow. But for Katelyn, despite all the care and love and attention, the change in her sister is devastating. "Before, it didn't feel like we were saying goodbye to Keira. It felt like we were just waiting for her to come back to us. Dad said she wouldn't be the same when she came back, but I didn't believe him. When I saw her, I started crying because she didn't look the same. She looked like she was dead."

———

Grief, as nurses know better than anyone, is the form love takes when someone dies. Perhaps grief hurts as much as it ought to—as much and as fiercely as the person who has died was loved. On the day on which Keira donated her organs, nothing could have saved eleven-year-old Katelyn, twelve-year-old Keely, seven-year-old Bradley, Joe and Loanna from the agony of losing their sister, their daughter. Keira was too young, too vibrant, too loving, too vivacious, too brimming with hope and potential to die. Everyone in the Bristol Royal Hospital for Children strove to do their utmost to soften the blow, while knowing their attempts would be futile. Yet perhaps they showed a grieving family something else instead. That no matter how little time a person has left—or even if their death defies the ongoing beat of their heart—a human being still has value. A human being still deserves our love and care. If we live on past our deaths in the minds of those who love us—and isn't this the only kind of legacy, in the end, that counts?—then perhaps the staff in Bristol created memories that would, in time, far from now, bring comfort to a grieving family by reminding them how very much they cared.

———

On June 29, 2017, Mrs. Leach had given her Year Five class an end-of-year challenge. A primary school teacher in the Devon village of South Molton, she asked the children to imagine returning in September for the new school year. *What are your hopes for Year Six?* she asked them. *What do you want to try really hard at?* She told them to write it all down in a letter that they would open in the autumn, to remind them of what they wanted to achieve. With their heads bent over their desks, the children set to work. One of them was Keira. She addressed herself by her nickname, Bob, then handed her letter to Mrs. Leach. The letters remained in a drawer throughout the long summer holiday. Only at the start of the new term, a month after Keira's death, did Mrs. Leach remember they were there. She took Keira's letter, unopened, to Joe and Loanna. In the careful rounded handwriting beloved of young girls, they read the following words:

Dear Bob,
Over the next year I would like to get better at writing.
Get better at looking after animals.
Get better at English.
I will do my best to achieve them.

Byeeeeeeeeee!
Yours sincerely,
Keira

Transplant

"If I do one job well, it is stopping bleeding. That is the essence of my expertise—I control bleeding. When I get called by other surgeons for help when things go wrong, it's because they know I can stop the bleeding. I see the lifeblood running out, literally, and I stop it." It has taken cardiothoracic surgeon Asif Hasan decades of operating on open hearts to acquire his particular superpower, and on August 2, 2017, his skill was tested once more.

Max lay on the table, his sternum sawn in two, the retractor's teeth applied. Gloved hands cranked at stainless steel—it takes brute force to prize a rib cage apart. Max's heart, once exposed, was slack and gargantuan, smacking feebly like a fish on a deck. A travesty of a heart, in truth, not so much beating as floundering. Without the LVAD, it was abundantly clear, Max would have died long ago. Yet unlike the poignancy of the theater in Bristol, where the surgeons were working in the shadow of death, here in Newcastle the stage was set for hope, for the possibility of life restored.

Initially, consultant Fabrizio De Rita led the surgery. As everyone had suspected, over the preceding six months, the titanium pump—so vital for sustaining the flow of blood through Max's body—had adhered to the myocardium, causing severe inflammation and scarring that now encased the entire heart. The fusion of muscle, scar, and metal was proving fiendishly difficult to disentangle. Fabrizio labored away at the scar tissue, but as the dissection wore on, his concerns grew. He called his mentor, Asif, for backup. "It was logical for Asif to assist me," says Fabrizio. "I was a relatively new consultant, and he had many more years of experience than me. Plus, he'd been pioneering these sorts of procedures not only in Newcastle, but also across the entire European community. From a technical point of view, his expertise was invaluable. Also," he adds, alluding to the era of 1960s heart surgeon superstars, "these days we all recognize that working together with four hands is much better than working alone."

Like Fabrizio, Asif takes a dim view of surgeons who hunger for individual glory. "Teamwork is what matters. You can achieve so much if you don't care who takes the credit. In transplant, credit is shared between the cardiologists, the nurses, the anesthesiologists, everyone. Who would want all the glory? Glory would be like having a sword of Damocles hanging over you, and when it does fall, there is no glory in any of this. You are responsible for a child's life. The responsibility is constantly there, you can never get away from it. You are always beholden to this inner feeling that if something goes wrong, it was you. So when you operate, you have to try and not worry about what has happened in the past—and remember that the future is another country. Just exist in the moment."

Asif's NHS office is the tattered embodiment of precisely these attitudes. Dingy, cramped, and in dire need of new paint and furniture, he has happily shared it for years with another surgeon, when he could easily have pulled rank and demanded his own, something glitzier and more befitting a surgical superstar. He did not. Instead, one of the most renowned transplant surgeons in Europe flops down for middle-of-the-night catnaps in between surgeries on a sofa so threadbare it looks like it may have been nibbled by mice, sustained by Nescafé and an industrial-sized tin of Coffee-Mate sitting on his bookshelves. The trappings of status and power are of no interest to

Asif, whose idea of an exotic vacation is visiting orchards containing rare breeds of apples, and who is described by one of his cardiology colleagues as "simply unique and altruistic. He is always the last one standing. He'll walk into an operation when someone else is tired and finish off for them. He'll let the juniors go while he stays to the end. He doesn't say to the junior, 'You close.' He says, 'I'll close and you go.' He's just as happy doing the mundane stuff as he is doing the impressive stuff. He will be there at three o'clock in the morning, checking on things, making sure that the patient is safe."

When Fabrizio called Asif to say he was worried about the impact of the scarring on his surgical field, Asif did not hesitate to come in. "Of course I did—because if you hit something while you're dissecting out the LVAD, you can lose everything very quickly at that point." It was a prophetic understatement. By pure chance, what happened next was recorded live by a BBC film crew who happened to be in theater, making a documentary about the fiftieth anniversary of Christiaan Barnard's first heart transplant.[1] First, the BBC cameras captured Asif's dismay at the extent of the scarring. "This heart is just completely stuck everywhere," you hear him mutter from behind his surgical mask, hands deep in Max's chest cavity. "There is no anatomical demarcation. We can't see anything. It's like cement. Basically we're trying to peel off cement and get to see the heart beneath without damaging the heart or the device itself. That's the challenge."[2] The carapace of scar tissue had effectively blindfolded the surgeons. Asif and Fabrizio were in the dark, instinctively groping with razor-sharp blades and a red-hot diathermy probe, while knowing that one false stroke could be fatal. "It is touch and feel—you feel pressure, something pulsing, something not," says Fabrizio, with Asif adding on camera: "What we try and do is find areas of the heart we can recognize. It's archaeology, digging. Your senses are heightened, all of them are tuned in. The sense you don't want to use is your hearing because if you get audible bleeding, you're in real trouble."

With the deft strokes of Renaissance artisans, the pair had finally addressed the bulk of the adhesions. Confident they were nearly there, Asif asked Alison Davidson, the transplant coordinator with them in theater, to call the surgeons waiting beside Keira in Bristol. At 5:41 p.m., Alison told Keira's team they could cross-clamp the aorta. A few minutes later, the Bristol team called back. The aorta was cross-clamped and the clock was ticking. Four hours maximum in which to dispatch a heart across three hundred miles, extract it from its bed of ice, deposit it safely into Asif's and Fabrizio's hands, *and* allow them to flawlessly stitch each great vessel into place so that warm fresh blood could at last replenish tissues in dire need of oxygen.

For those rare individuals with the temerity to take their scalpels to our fragile hearts, timing is everything. Only rarely will a transplant surgeon authorize the removal of a heart before their own preparatory dissection of the recipient's chest is complete or very close to completion. Otherwise the risk is too great of an unexpected delay causing irreversible damage to the donor heart. Fabrizio explains: "If we are opening a chest for the very first time, it may only take us about ten minutes before we are ready to accept the donor heart. So sometimes the heart is out and on its way to us before we start. But if the patient has had heart surgery before, we know there will be scarring and it could take much longer. We have to minimize the time that the donor heart stays in the box. If the heart arrives and I'm not ready to implant it as soon as possible, then I am wasting time. *I* would rather be the one waiting, not the heart, so I say, 'Well, look, the patient is safe on the table, everything is ready and open and dissected now, so they can wait. Let's take a break.'"

It is not uncommon in a heart transplant for the entire surgical team to scrub out and decamp to a break room for coffee, leaving the patient anesthetized on the table with their ribs retracted and heart exposed, the gaping wound cursorily draped in plastic. "Say the patient is being operated on for the fifth time, we might get inside the chest and spend the next two hours fighting the adhesions and getting things free. If the heart arrives too early, you're not ready practically, you're not ready mentally," says Fabrizio. "Your mind keeps saying, 'Okay, the heart is here now, it's in the box, we must take it out now.' That sets off a spiral of feelings that might lead to wrong decisions, because you're not focused on what you need to do. So no—just get yourself safely into the chest, dissect the heart out, and then you can wait as much as you want."

On this occasion, there was no respite. Six thousand feet in the air and hurtling forward at two hundred miles per hour, a human heart in a box was bisecting Britain. And this uncanny flight—this preposterous dislocation of a heart in orbit—kept Asif and Fabrizio toiling to free Max's heart from every last adhesion. Deep within his opened chest, at last the structures were appearing more clearly, like trees emerging from a fog in winter. Asif had just enough time to make out the aorta when, without warning, a scarlet arc of arterial blood gushed across the surgical field. In seconds, the chest cavity was awash with blood. Asif's white gloves were spattered crimson. He had accidentally sliced into Max's pulmonary artery. "Uh-oh," he murmured, betraying no hint of anxiety. "Please get me a swab, thank you." Asif jammed his finger into the hole he had made. The pulsing blood abated. "Get me a suture, please," he requested politely. Clipped, calm, precise instructions, exactly what a team craves in a crisis. The room looked on, aghast, spellbound, as Asif arrested a bloodbath with the finger of one hand, while fighting with the digits of the other to place a stitch in an artery already drowned in blood.

———

The *Oxford Dictionary of Philosophy* defines the meaning of "courage" with precision and elegance:

> An action is courageous if it is an attempt to achieve an end
> despite penalties, risks, costs, or difficulties of sufficient gravity
> to deter most people. Similarly a state such as cheerfulness
> is courageous if it is sustained in spite of such difficulties.
> A courageous person is characteristically able to attempt
> such actions or maintain such states. For Aristotle, courage
> is dependent on sound judgement, for it needs to be known
> whether the end justifies the risk incurred. Similarly, courage is
> not the absence of fear (which may be a vice), but the ability to
> feel the appropriate amount of fear; courage is a mean between
> timidity and overconfidence.[3]

This definition could be a job description for the defining qualities of a heart surgeon. Which of us would dare to run the gauntlet of an opened heart? To inhabit by choice a blood-soaked world in which the life of a nine-year-old boy hangs on whether you can stop your fingers trembling?

There is, then, something beautifully apt about the etymology of "courage," which can be traced back to the Latin word *cor*, meaning "heart." Pioneering heart surgeons such as Christiaan Barnard are easy to castigate for recklessness, but they were also the living embodiment of the very thing they dared to cut into. It was then—and it remains today—courage that sets them apart from us. In 1956, for example, Barnard faced an eerily similar predicament to that in which Asif Hasan found himself now. Yet, unlike Asif, Barnard was only in his first year of learning open-heart surgery at the time, under the guidance of the renowned American surgeon Clarence Walton Lillehei. His role was not even to open the heart, but simply to prepare it for Lillehei's arrival in theater. The patient, a child of seven years, had a ventricular septal defect—a hole between the two ventricles of his heart—which Lillehei would be suturing shut on bypass.

With the boy's father watching him from above in a viewing gallery, Barnard opened the child's chest and looped surgical tape around the superior vena cava, ready to hook it up to the heart-lung machine. So far, so good. But while dissecting out the inferior vena cava, he instructed his assistant to cut into a piece of tissue blocking his path to the blood vessel. "Blood spurted out as though driven by a pump—and, indeed, it was a pump: we had cut into the heart," Barnard wrote in his autobiography.[4] Horrified, he tried to clamp the hole, but tore it further, and in seconds the heart was submerged in blood. Someone ran for Lillehei, while Barnard rummaged blindly to find the hole, only to feel the heartbeat growing fainter and fainter until the organ stopped in his hands. Lillehei managed to put the child on bypass to repair the laceration, but was unable to restart the heart. The boy was dead. Beneath the gaze of the father, unable to meet his eye, Barnard sutured shut the chest of the child he had just killed.

Asif confirms that the potential for tragedy in heart surgery is every bit as painful as its successes are intoxicating. "Nothing matches being in the zone in theater. But then it is equally matched by how bad it is if things are going wrong. When death occurs, when it all goes wrong, it just crashes down on one person, and that person is you. There is no escaping it; it is your mistake. You just killed that child. There really are no mitigating circumstances. So you can get really high, but also really low. The bottom line is you have to take both, the success and the failure. You have to tell yourself that you did not cause the disease. You did your best at that point in time. Your best wasn't good enough. But if you learn from it, this is all you can do."

Late that evening, Barnard sought out Lillehei to apologize for his lethal mistake. Lillehei was supportive, saying he, too, had made the same error:

> The only thing you can do is learn by your mistake. The next time you have bleeding, remember you can stop it by putting your finger in the hole. That gives you time to prepare and consolidate yourself, to get calm and think of what you have to do. . . . So tomorrow, go ahead and open the next patient's chest. We'll do the same thing. You go in and loop the vena cava and I'll wait for you.

The following day, Barnard was petrified. Lillehei stayed away from the theater until the very last moment. Upon arriving, he peered into the chest and nodded approvingly. "Good job," he told Barnard, and together they set to work.

———

As he stood with his finger plugging the hole in Max's pulmonary artery, Asif was icily calm. He knew exactly what he needed to do and how to do it. With his needle poised and a thread of surgical silk snaking across his blood-spattered glove, Asif's fingers moved with a mind of their own. "I have been in that position many, many times. Of course your heart rate will go up a little bit, but you're just in that moment, you know how you're going to deal with it. It's like when Andy Murray is playing, or Nadal, or something like that, you know? If they're sitting back on the baseline, their body knows what it's going to do. They're not going to succeed all of the time, but most of the time they will. They are already running in the right direction before the opponent has even hit the ball." Ignoring the blood that swamped his surgical field, Asif placed the first suture in the torn artery with the apparent insouciance of someone darning a sock. Deftly, he placed a second suture. Still using only one hand, he asked courteously for a tiny white Dacron patch that he then teased inside the pulmonary artery and coolly stitched into place. As abruptly as it started, the bleeding stopped. "People have said to me, 'How do you know? How can you see through red blood?' But because you have done it so many times, you know where the needle is going to come out. You drop it underneath the blood, but you know it will be in the right spot, the needle will be there, and you will find it, and it will come out where you know it will. It's that degree of technical muscle memory."

While Asif and Fabrizio resumed their dissection, Alison Davidson received an urgent call. Keira's heart had arrived. She left the operating theater to meet the paramedics in the ambulance bay. There, they handed over the blue plastic cooler that could easily have been packed with cans of lager. Alison wheeled the box into theater just after Max had been placed on the heart-lung machine. But Asif and Fabrizio were still struggling to free his heart from its adhesions. They had misjudged the timings of the surgeries, prematurely telling the surgical team in Bristol that they could cross-clamp the aorta when, in fact, they were nowhere near dissecting out Max's LVAD. "We're not ready for the heart yet," said Asif bluntly. It was the first moment in theater that any tension was palpable.

The pair continued to carve and burn—this controlled obliteration of an open chest—as there on the floor, plonked beside a waste bin filled with soiled tissues, sat the box that they hoped would transform death into life. Wielding his scalpel with renewed assertiveness, Asif instructed Fabrizio to do likewise: "When you come to this stage, you have to have the instincts of a cage fighter." There was no time to lose. If the delay lasted much longer, the pristine tissues of Keira's heart would move beyond the point of irreversible decline, putting Max's life in the balance.

———

Max's parents, Emma and Paul, had been waiting for this moment for 196 days, the duration of Max's placement on the list for a heart transplant. They had feared many times he would never reach it. As soon as Emma was told a match had been found, she called Paul at home in Cheshire. "It was very quiet when the phone rang," says Paul. "Emma said, 'He's got one, he's got one, he's got one, you need to get here straightaway!' I just remember it was like a dam bursting. When I put the phone down, I burst into tears. I couldn't help myself. There was no warning. A feeling I couldn't control had been building, building, building, and all of a sudden that emotion was released, the gratitude and the relief and the fear. I looked up to the heavens to say thank you, because I knew immediately that this was happening because another family was in an awful situation. Something horrendous had happened to them, but they had said yes. I thought of them straightaway because I felt so guilty." Through his tears, Paul spoke the words "I'm scared" out loud into the empty house. He knew there was a 25 percent chance Max would not survive the surgery, yet he had no better chance at life.

Just prior to the news of a donor, the BBC film crew had asked Max how he felt about waiting for a new heart. "Every day I've got that nervous feeling," Max answered. "Say you were going to go sky-diving, I get that nervous sensation, in case it comes. Like, 'Will it happen? Is this the day?'"[5] When asked what he would do when he received his new heart, a slow smile crept across Max's face before he blurted: "Annoy my brother! Prank my granny and grandpa!" In fact, Max had privately reached the point where at times he didn't care if he lived or died. The quality of his life had been so poor for so long that the prospect of a transplant, once so terrifying, had ceased even to concern him. "I was just at the point where I thought, 'You know, I'll be stuck in here forever until I die,'" he says. "It's like I was waiting to go. I was at the end. I was getting really frustrated, like I was jealous of other kids. Because you could see the park across the way where kids were playing football. I just wanted to be doing that, too."

That afternoon, Max, Harry, Emma, and Paul sat quietly chatting inside his cubicle, trying to distract him from the imminent surgery. "The nurses let me put my music on loud, probably because they thought I could die," says Max. "Thinking about it now, it's quite sad, you know? I gave my dad a hug and my brother a hug. I knew inside I could probably die from the operation. But it's so weird, I wasn't scared. I knew I could die, but when you actually come to facing it, you just kind of accept it. You think, 'Well, okay, fine.' I suppose I was also excited, thinking, 'If this does go well, I'm free. I can do what I want again.'"

Once he had been given his pre-medications, Max became manic and emotionally disinhibited, lurching erratically from laughter to tears. As he was wheeled toward the theater, singing and flailing, his parents tried to calm him down. After all the agonizing months of waiting, suddenly time was racing, flying, and Paul and Emma could not keep up. Too quickly the doors of the theater loomed, the portal to the jarring world of iodine and masks, steel and drapes, and the oppressive pall of fear. A box on the floor was filled with bags of blood labeled with the name "Max Johnson." When she saw them—a snapshot of the violence to come—it was all Emma could do not to keel over. A form of courage of her own kept her standing, the might with which she loved her child. She and Paul had been here once before, inside the pandemonium of a theater poised for open-heart surgery, but that did not ease their terror. "I kept thinking, 'This is different to before. This time they are going to cross a point of no return. If something goes wrong, that will be it. It is either going to work, or my boy is going to die,'" says Paul.

Just before his anesthetic, Max grew quiet, as though trying to fathom the monitors, equipment, and faces in masks towering above him. He began to whimper, wide-eyed with fear, before a moment of eerie lucidity. "I wanted to make sure that my parents knew I loved them," he recalls. "You know, I wanted to make sure this was a really nice goodbye, because I could die. I remember my dad behind my bed, stroking my head. And if I think about it, he was probably scared, too, because he was probably thinking I could die as well." Barely audible above the cacophony of the theater, the last words Max said to his mum and dad were: "It will be a while until I see you again, I love you both." "We love you, too," they sobbed back at him, but Max was already drifting into unconsciousness.

———

It is not called a theater for nothing. Spotlights converged from above on Asif, as his performance approached its denouement. After the slog of the dissection, the drama of the arterial hemorrhage, the suspense of the emergency repair, he could not resist a moment of playing to the crowd. He tugged Max's heart out of his chest, titanium pump still attached, and glanced briefly at the shattered tissue before dumping it unceremoniously in a plastic bowl. Without giving the ruined organ a backward glance, he held the bowl out sideways for someone to take from him as he growled dismissively, "Throw it in the bin."

This was the point of no return, the hinterland that so horrified Paul, the void where his son's heart once resided. A humming, whirring mechanical oxygenator now performed the role of Max's heart and lungs. Crimson laced with Prussian blue in, vivid cherry red out again. His entire circulation flowed through the twists and coils and convolutions of the heart-lung machine under the vigilant eye of the perfusionist. It was a miracle of modern technology that looked more like a mangled Pompidou Center. Flick a switch, and Max would die. A life outsourced to pumps and tubing: it was too outlandish to grasp.

The stage, at last, was set for Keira. Only she could resurrect this boy whose life was all but over. And here—now—before our eyes, it appears, a second miracle, this marvel of a human heart in deepest hibernation. A theater nurse prizes the lid from the cooler and sweeps away a coat of ice chips. Cold diffuses through latex into flesh as she plunges her gloved hands into crushed ice. Triple-bagged, submerged in fluid, a perfect yet petrified living organ, Keira's heart, Max's hope, rising now from its frozen bed, wondrous and incomprehensible.

Asif is calling for steroids from the operating table. He and Fabrizio are almost ready to transplant the heart, which, from the moment Max's blood begins to flow through its tissues, will be under attack from his immune system. T cells and B cells, lymphocytes and phagocytes—all of them doing their vicious best to destroy the heart they see as a foreign invasion. For Max to live, these cells must be suppressed. The massive dose of interoperative steroids will act, Asif says, "like a hydrogen bomb—it kills everything."

It is time. Asif lifts Keira's heart as though it might bolt from his grasp if startled. Every eye is glued to the hands that clasp the promise of life for the boy on the table. This isn't medicine, it's witchcraft. Asif places the heart in the empty cavern of the opened chest. His wrists disappear inside Max's body and, together with Fabrizio, he begins to stitch. Two adults and two children are briefly one, four people sharing the same shell of a body. Slowly, methodically, the surgeons suture severed aorta to severed aorta, severed vena cava to severed vena cava. Each great vessel is married to its mirror part, Keira to Max, Max to Keira. It is the neatest, most uniform, most precise needlework: Alexis Carrel would be nodding his approval. And while they sew, the surgeons know, a secret alchemy is underway. Keira's heart is becoming warmer. Dozily, dreamily, her myocardial cells are waking up, becoming a little more metabolically active. More than anything, this heart aches to beat. Honed by millennia of evolution, it exists with one aim alone, a single-minded thirst for pumping. As the temperature rises, the mitochondria twitch and the tiniest of electrical impulses flicker uncertainly across dormant myocardium. Imperceptibly for now, far too weak to force a contraction, but growing, building, strengthening. The electricity, says Asif, is what "makes the magic happen," and slowly but surely—before fresh blood has even found this emptied organ—the magic has begun. There is a quiver, a shudder, a microscopic gyration. No blood, no oxygen, just the merest hint of warmth, and already Keira's heart is trying to beat. This is not a "good" heart, as the surgeons said in Bristol, this is a glorious heart, one of the wonders of the world, an earthly miracle. Infinitely more spectacular than some minor lunar footstep, this heart wipes the floor with human engineering. Heart of hearts, Max's lifeline, the purest love gift, a marvel on the brink of beating.

Asif unclamps Max's great vessels. His circulation is now united with that of the heart-lung machine. For the first time in over four hours, warm oxygenated blood flows through the four starved chambers of Keira's heart. You imagine its cells as creatures deranged with relief, falling on the oxygen, devouring it. It is life itself that is being transferred. First from Max's blood to the parched cells of Keira's heart, and then from the heart back into Max's parched tissues, the liver, the kidneys, the eyes, the brain, all for so long denied a proper blood supply. The quivers—fibrillations—now swiftly resolve into recognizable contractions. Keira's heart, now Max's heart, is moving, beating, in an unfamiliar chest, tethered to unfamiliar vessels. A century of medical innovation has brought us to this, the most brilliant minds, the most audacious hands, the most unfettered imaginations. Asif's and Fabrizio's eyes bore into their handiwork, searching for evidence of leakage. Not a trickle, not a drop, the anastomoses are perfect. They watch and wait, cautious, hypervigilant, giving the heart ample time to recover before daring to attempt to take Max off bypass.

Finally, they ask the perfusionist to gradually dial down the support Max receives from the heart-lung machine. Three-quarters and then wait; half and then wait; a quarter and then wait; and then—nothing. All eyes on the heart, nobody breathing. It is pumping now without any external assistance and Max's blood pressure seems to be stable. Asif stares into the chest with his hawklike intensity, not taking his eyes off the heart for a millisecond. "You can only relax when the heart is completely off the heart-lung machine, because that is the proof you must have—is this heart capable of pumping the blood around the body?" he says. Five, ten, fifteen minutes elapse. Still Asif waits, watches. Still the blood pressure holds. Finally, he nods at Fabrizio to release the retractor and slowly, tectonically, the battered ribs begin to ease back into place, shrouding once more the crypt of Max's chest, the vault in which Keira's heart has been laid to rest.

Aftermath

The day after Max's transplant—eight months since he was first admitted to the hospital—Emma cannot stop looking at his cheeks. "They were pink, he was pink. I'd not seen him like that for nearly a year. I'd forgotten what it looked like. I was so used to that pale face and now his cheeks were pink again. And that was the moment when I thought, 'he's been injected with life from another person.' I started to think, 'My God, I wonder what actually happened?'" Max's vivacity prompts Emma to ask the doctors if anything is known about the donor. They can say only that the donor was "age-appropriate," but the words contain multitudes. "I nodded slowly because I was taking in that the donor must have been nine. That was the tipping point, the moment when I started to really think about how the heart had reached Max. I felt overwhelmed with gratitude to whoever that family was, because they had made Max's cheeks pink when they could have been blue, if it had gone the other way. They had saved him."

Within three or four days, Max's cheeks are plump as well as flushed, since he can finally process food again. His vision, which had been blurred, rapidly improves once his retinas are no longer starved of oxygen. He is chatty, ebullient, full of sparkle. A week after the transplant, the nurses don't know whether to cheer or restrain him when suddenly he sets off at a run down a corridor. The

BBC film crew returns to ask Max how he feels about his new heart, and he answers: "In the morning I say good morning to it and I send it all the love I can, so it settles in. I'm trying to give it a nice new home in a new body. Just the biggest thank-you to whoever gave it to me because they saved my life."

The greatest threat for Max initially is that of hyperacute rejection. In this rare complication of a transplant, the recipient's blood contains preexisting antibodies that recognize and attack the donor organ, causing catastrophic damage. Screening for antibodies prior to transplant usually ensures none are present, but very occasionally the screen may miss them. Hyperacute rejection has a 70 percent mortality rate and Max's cardiologists monitor him exceptionally closely.[1]

Asif, meanwhile, has redirected his focus onto the children on the ward who still need open-heart surgery. It is another example of the extreme compartmentalization without which he knows he could not survive in his job. With typical self-deprecation, he describes his involvement with his patients: "When the children come in, I'm the bus driver who simply picks them up from one point and drops them off at the other. During that journey I am completely responsible for them. I need to make sure that the tires are okay, there's petrol in the engine, the seats are clean, and they are safe. But when I drop them off, my job is done. I'm not responsible for what happens to them afterwards and I wasn't responsible beforehand, either. The disease is in them, it's not in me. You have to accept that you didn't cause any of this. These children are very sick and sometimes they do die. You have to do the same operation today when yesterday a child died from that operation. You can't be emotionally stuck with what happened before. You have to physically and mentally delete it, cut and paste, clear your mind. It's not easy. But you have to restart and refocus."

Either Paul or Emma arrives on the ward each morning at eight o'clock sharp to prepare and administer Max's immunosuppressants. The responsibility feels immense and daunting. Although Max has survived the immediate threat of hyperacute rejection, without these drugs his body could reject his new heart at any time. In order to build up their confidence in supervising his medication regime at home, Emma and Paul lay out the drugs on the hospital tray themselves— cyclosporine, prednisolone, azathioprine, aciclovir. For the rest of his life, Max will need to take precisely timed, twice-daily doses of cyclosporine, or an equivalent drug, to prevent his body from rejecting his heart. When Emma looks at the rows of capsules, she can't believe these little pills are all that is keeping her son alive.

———

Ever since the early days of organ transplantation in the 1960s, doctors and their patients have been walking a tightrope between the destructive potency of the immune system and the perils of suppressing it. Back then, the only drugs that weakened the immune system sufficiently for a patient to tolerate their new transplanted organ also left the patient vulnerable to overwhelming infection from viruses or bacteria. Then, in 1969, a drug was unearthed—literally—that would change everything.[2] The Swiss pharmaceutical company Sandoz had set up a quixotic program for discovering new drugs in which they asked their employees to collect soil samples from other countries whenever they went traveling.[3] Sandoz had been inspired by the ad hoc nature in which scientists had previously stumbled across other groundbreaking drugs, such as Alexander Fleming's discovery of penicillin after a *Penicillium* mold spore randomly contaminated one of his lab cultures. Once back in the Sandoz lab, the assorted soil samples were screened for fungal metabolites in case they possessed antibacterial, antifungal, immunosuppressive, or anticancer properties—and could therefore form the basis of revolutionary new drugs.

Every week, around twenty samples of random soil from around the world were delivered to the Sandoz lab. One of them—sample 24-556 from an employee on vacation in Norway—showed startling immunosuppressive qualities.[4] Named after its cyclical structure and its derivation from fungal spores, the new drug, cyclosporine A, began to be tested on humans in 1978. The results were extraordinary. One-year survival rates after transplantation soared from 32 to 70 percent for liver patients and from 54 to 77 percent for kidney patients.[5] In 1983, cyclosporine was approved by the US Food and Drug Administration for use in kidney, liver, and heart transplants. The production process, memorably described by the *New York Times*, seems not dissimilar to industrial-scale potion-brewing in a witch's cauldron: "[Cyclosporine] is produced through a fermentation process. The fungus is grown in stainless-steel containers. The compound is then extracted from the fungus and put into a broth, which is purified to remove contaminants."[6]

Cyclosporine revolutionized transplant medicine. Although the drug was in no sense benign—it caused renal failure in some patients and increased their risk of developing cancer—researchers found that it was highly selective in suppressing a particular cell of the immune system known as the helper T cell. Unlike all the immunosuppressants to date, cyclosporine specifically prevented the activation of T cells, while leaving other parts of the immune system unaffected. It was therefore able to minimize the chances of rejection, while leaving a large part of the body's defenses against infection intact. Thanks to cyclosporine, transplant recipients could reasonably hope to live for years—decades, even—without succumbing to a fatal infection.

Line by line, wire by wire, Max is slowly detached from the various tubes, drips, and pumps, the paraphernalia of the critically ill that has surrounded him for the best part of a year. Scott House provides a nearby transplant flat precisely to help ease families into living independently again. One day, Max is judged sufficiently stable to make the move into the flat. Next, the family ventures farther afield, on a day trip to a local beach, where Max experiences the dizzy delights of paddling in the waves with his brother. On September 14, just six weeks after his operation, he is told he is well enough to go home. "How can you begin to thank the team who had so skillfully saved your son's life and given him a second chance at life?" says Paul. "Without exception, they'd proven that their chosen career was, at its very heart, a true vocation. They'd gone out of their way to make Max's time in hospital as comfortable and pain-free as possible, both physically and psychologically. Wonderful people doing an incredible job. Thank you, thank you, thank you."

At 4:30 p.m., Emma's car pulls up outside their old farmworker's cottage in Winsford, Cheshire. Sitting in the front passenger seat, radiating excitement, is Max, a boy who has spent a ninth of his life not at home but in hospital. As soon as Harry sees him, he flings his arms around his brother, gripping him as though his life depends on it. The brothers stand in an embrace that lasts an age. Then Harry leads Max to his bedroom. When Max had been at his lowest ebb in the hospital, Paul and Emma had tried to lift his spirits by encouraging him to write a wish list of all the things he looked forward to doing once he had a new heart. The list Max compiled was heartbreakingly unambitious: seeing his friends again, climbing a tree, playing with his brother in the back garden. At the top of the list was something Paul has been secretly working on for many weeks to achieve, all the while knowing that Max might never leave the hospital alive to see it: a new bedroom. When Max opens the door of his redecorated bedroom, it still smells of fresh paint. There are new bunk beds, disco lights, speakers, and—pride of place in the center of the room—his grandfather's vintage turntable, now professionally refurbished. Truly this is kit for next-level DJing, and Max's smile could light up a small planet.

Max ends his first day at home with his family curled up in his father's lap in his new bedroom. They have been listening to music together, admiring the sound that only vinyl can generate through classic KEF speakers. Max's eyelids droop and he allows his head to fall against the warmth and security of his father's chest. It is an ordinary scene, quotidian and familiar, being replayed in homes across the country. Yet during the long months of transplant-list purgatory, whenever Paul allowed himself to imagine a moment like this, he berated himself for his self-indulgence, for wallowing in fantasy. This humdrum image has been sneaked past death and snatched from oblivion. And all that his son may go on to experience, the wash of the ocean, the smell of freshly cut grass, the thrill of a first kiss, the taste of Mum's roast potatoes—all the myriad moments that make life worth living—will always and forever have been enabled by Keira, the girl who gave her heart to a dying boy that he might, for a time, share its marching beat and bask in its boundless vitality.

———

Asif Hasan is very clear about who matters most in organ transplantation—and it is certainly not himself as the surgeon. "I have always believed that the greatest credit for what we do in transplant must go to the donor, to the gift which was given either by the donor or the donor family. Nothing else can happen without the donor. A family has—in the midst of the most abysmal circumstances—made a decision to think about others. It is remarkable, it is astonishing."

Having first decided to donate Keira's organs, Joe and Loanna continue endeavoring to construct meaning and goodness from the wreckage of life without their daughter. Even while blasted by grief, they set up a small charity, Inspired by Keira, to raise awareness of the importance of organ donation and to support other families confronting the sudden loss of a child.

Shortly after Max arrives home, Emma sits down to compose the most difficult letter she has ever written. She and Paul try to find the words with which to thank the family, nameless and faceless, of the child whose heart beats in Max. "We wanted to capture our feeling of gratitude, but also recognize their loss," says Emma. "I just tried to write from the heart by imagining myself in the shoes of the person who had lost a child. What would I have liked to receive? What would be sensitive wording? What would bring comfort?" Paul adds his words to Emma's first draft, and together they read it out loud to Max and Harry. It feels, or so they imagine, to be an act of closure:

> Even in your grief, you have made a selfless decision to help others and we are indescribably grateful to you. . . . We wanted you to know that your sacrifice was not in vain and you have given an incredible legacy of love and good will to others. We thank you so much for making a decision that has saved our son and given him the prospect of a future ahead of him. As he grows older, we will encourage him to cherish his heart in memory of you. With our eternal gratitude . . .

As per the strict rules governing contact between donor and recipient families after a transplant, Paul and Emma are permitted to use only their first names in their letter, which is sent to Joe

212 The Story *of a* Heart

and Loanna via the intermediary of NHS Blood and Transplant. Ordinarily, these precautions protect families from the potentially traumatic experience of discovering each other's identities. In Max's case, however, a detailed account of his story has already appeared on the front pages of a national newspaper. Even before Keira's family receives Paul and Emma's letter, they have been led by the media coverage to suspect that her heart may have been given to Max, a boy the same age as she was, and who received his transplant around the time that Keira's organs were retrieved. As soon as Loanna opens the letter and sees the names Max, Emma, Paul, and Harry, her theory is confirmed. She searches online for the *Mirror* articles and there finds Max, vivacious, impish, the contours of his chest framing her own daughter's heart. It is both wondrous and incomprehensible, taking weeks for her to begin to process—but a seed is planted and begins to grow.

One day, nearly three months after Max's transplant, the family is packing to go away on a short family vacation when Emma quickly checks her Facebook page. She grows so quiet and still while staring at the screen that Paul is alarmed something terrible has happened. "What's the matter, love?" he asks, and Emma bursts into tears. The private message she has just received is from Loanna. It reads: "I think you may have our daughter's heart and it's the most beautiful heart in the world."

"I felt shock, excitement, trepidation, and anxiety all rolled into one," says Emma. She and Paul embark on a tentative series of exchanges with Loanna on Facebook. "We were desperate not to say anything that could cause offense or overstep the mark," says Paul. "We were conscious of how raw their grief must still be." One day, Loanna asks Emma if she and Paul would like to see a photo of Keira. Her face appears on Emma's phone, radiating beauty and kindness. "It was like being hit in the solar plexus," says Paul. "You're looking at the smiling face of the little girl who died. You look at her chest and think, 'The heart in that chest is now in our son's chest.' This amazing little girl who was their everything is now no longer there. It was wonderful, but also very, very difficult to see."

Perhaps inevitably after Loanna's first message to Emma, the two families begin to discuss the idea of meeting. Emma and Paul are initially hesitant, concerned about causing Joe and Loanna unintended pain. They fear that Max's milestones to come—reaching his tenth birthday, starting secondary school, becoming a teenager—might be harrowing reminders of everything Keira has been denied. In fact, both Joe and Loanna derive enormous comfort from knowing that some of Keira still exists within Max. "There is a part of her who lives on, it's as simple as that," says Loanna.

In May 2018, nine months after Max's transplant, Keira's entire family travels to Cheshire to meet the Johnsons at home. Like Paul and Emma, Joe and Loanna know that the public is likely to be captivated by the heartwarming consequences of their decision to donate Keira's organs, and all this has meant to both families. It is a valuable opportunity to raise awareness of organ donation. The families agree to let Jeremy Armstrong from the *Mirror* attend the meeting. The story he writes is deeply moving. "Max reminds me so much of my daughter," says Loanna in her interview. "He is always smiling, a bouncy little boy, and that is exactly how she was, the most loving, happy child. I see her in Max. I get such comfort knowing he is doing so well."[7]

The most heartrending moment of all occurs when Emma produces a stethoscope, borrowed from a friend, in case Keira's family would like to listen to her heart inside Max's chest. Laughing with disbelief and wonder, the children form an excited queue to hear their sister's heartbeat. Then it is the turn of Joe, the father who chose to surrender his daughter's heart to honor her abundance of kindness. It was Joe, selflessly, who signed the forms, who clasped Keira tight, who felt the last rays of warmth this heart ever gave to her, who set in motion the cascade of events that has brought us here, to this unfathomable point, where Max is pulling up his T-shirt, displaying his scar, giggling with Keely and Katelyn, while he, Joe, is staring at a little boy's chest, skinny, disfigured, and undulating visibly to the indefatigable beat of his daughter's heart, strong and beautiful, nestled deep beneath its barricade of ribs. Joe places the buds of the stethoscope in his ears and lays its drum on the skin of Max's chest. He takes a deep breath, and listens.

Epilogue

On May 20, 2020, after months of tireless campaigning by Max, Emma, Loanna, Paul, and Joe, the Organ Donation (Deemed Consent) Act was passed into English law. It was officially named on the statute books as Max and Keira's Law in recognition of the extraordinary role played by both children in raising awareness of the importance of organ donation.[1]

In the first year after the law was changed, 296 people in England donated their organs under the new opt-out system, nearly a third of the total number of 1,021 donations that took place that year.[2] The reverberations of Keira and her family's altruism continue to be felt every year in the form of the hundreds of additional patients whose lives are saved by the donor organs they might otherwise not have received.

There remains a desperate shortage of donor organs worldwide. In particular, the number of children globally who could benefit from a transplant vastly exceeds the number of available organs. In the UK, children in urgent need of a transplant continue to wait two and a half times as long as adults to receive an organ. At any one time, around two hundred children in Britain are waiting for a transplant, of whom around fifty need a new heart.[3] Around one in six of the children waiting for a donor heart continue to die while on the heart transplant list. Clinicians and scientists are working today with every bit as much passion and resolve as the early pioneers of transplant surgery in the twentieth century to increase the number of usable organs, prolong the time in which they can tolerate ischemia, and, in the future, perhaps even grow replacement organs from a patient's own stem cells, eliminating the need for immunosuppression after a transplant.[4]

A huge glass-doored display cabinet dominates Joe and Loanna's living room. An unabashedly effusive shrine to a child whose charm and ebullience captivated everyone, it contains an abundance of vivid pink and orange. You can see Keira's favorite clothes and sneakers, her most beloved soft toys, her gymkhana rosettes, the hard hat she wore when riding, her letters, drawings, doodles, certificates, and a galaxy of photos of that glorious smile, beaming mischief and joy at the camera. Sarah Crosby still visits regularly and will continue to do so for as long as they need her. "They are an exceptionally beautiful family. I am in awe of them. It is an absolute blessing to know them, and I am still amazed by their strength and generosity," she says.

Loanna continues working to raise awareness of organ donation, visiting schools in Devon to talk to classes about transplants. Not once has she encountered a child who did not wish to donate their organs after their death.

On May 12, 2022, the Ball family were overjoyed when Loanna gave birth to a baby girl, who has since grown into a beautiful toddler with her sister Keira's sky-blue eyes, honey-colored hair, and irresistibly infectious smile. Her name is Kyra-Mai. The Balls and the Johnsons remain in touch with each other, and Emma and Paul have been thrilled to watch Kyra-Mai grow and flourish.

Max, Emma, Paul, and Harry are living with the complicated knowledge that a person's life expectancy after receiving a heart transplant is on average only fourteen years. At the time of writing, Max has already lived for nearly half that time. He, like his parents, is putting his faith in the creativity and invention of medical science, remaining optimistic that solutions will be found to the innumerable risks and challenges of lifelong immunosuppression. He takes his medications religiously, fully aware of what could happen if he doesn't. Emma and Paul are learning not to quake too fearfully each time fifteen-year-old Max disappears into town with his mates, enjoying whatever it is that teenage boys enjoy getting up to, though always promising, in this post-pandemic world, to keep hand sanitizer in his pocket.

Throughout his brother's illness, Harry rarely confided his feelings. A quiet boy, self-contained and thoughtful, he absorbed it all silently, through eleven-year-old eyes, until one day, as he was approaching sixth form, he discovered that what he had witnessed during Max's months in the hospital had kindled within him an idea that persisted and began to crystallize. The science and technology behind his brother's heart transplant were inspiring in their own right, but what had really captivated Harry's imagination was the dedication and humanity of the doctors like Asif Hasan. Harry toiled furiously at his science A levels, while working in a nursing home on the weekends to learn firsthand the realities of caring for others. In September 2023, he began the first term of a medical degree at Newcastle University's School of Medicine.

Nothing was easy after Max came home. He struggled with severe insomnia and was diagnosed with post-traumatic stress syndrome caused by the multiple traumas he had experienced during his long months in hospital. He had missed a great deal of school, but worked hard to catch up and is now halfway through his GCSEs. Recently, he developed a love of fishing. On the weekends, he likes to sit with his dad on a quiet riverbank, surrounded by fresh air and birdsong, patiently waiting for a tug on the line. Occasionally they talk about his time in hospital. One day, Paul told Max about the period in his life when he was so critically unwell that his doctors and parents feared he could die at any time. With his heart, liver, and kidneys all failing simultaneously, every day had felt like running a gauntlet. "So it was like I was fighting with a hundred-pound carp on the end of a five-pound line?" Max said. "Yes," Paul replied. "Yes, it was. And that hundred-pound carp was your mortality, Max. You needed a miracle to win that battle." The sun was dipping low in the sky, and they decided to call it a day. Bathed in golden light that was both gleaming and dying, father and son retraced their steps along the bank. Fleetingly, the angle of the sun caught the water in such a way that an incandescence of reds, pinks, purples, and oranges poured from its surface. It was breathtaking, heart-stopping, spectacular, and then, in a moment, it was gone.

Acknowledgments

My heartfelt thanks to the Ball family—Loanna, Joe, Katelyn, Keely, Bradley, and Kyra-Mai—and the Johnson family—Emma, Paul, Max and Harry—for so generously and courageously sharing their story with me over many conversations. Thanks too to every one of the healthcare professionals who gave up their time to talk to me about their role in the journey of Keira's heart. I know how vary painful it sometimes was to relive those events as they unfolded, and I am immensely grateful to you all. NHS Blood and Transplant were incredibly supportive of this project, helping me check facts and understand important nuances of organ transplantation. Particular thanks to Suzi Browne.

I have been so lucky to be supported by the team at Scribner. Kara Watson, Nan Graham, Joie Asuquo, Laura Wise, Georgia Brainard, Colleen Nuccio, Jaya Miceli, Stu Smith, thank you so much for your vital roles in helping bring this book into being.

Emma and Paul Johnson wrote their own, beautiful version of their, Max's, and Keira's story, entitled *Golden Heart* and published in 2019. They kindly permitted me to draw on their own written words in the writing of this book.

So many friends and colleagues have helped me with their incisive feedback on, and discussions, about the book—thank you, all. And with this, as with all my books, my husband has been such a scrupulously honest, incisive, and candid first editor—giving me exactly the kind of early feedback a writer needs. Thank you, Dave, for absolutely everything.

Lastly, because she definitely deserves her own paragraph, I cannot sing from the rooftops too loudly about the kindness and brilliance of my friend and agent, Clare Alexander. You are wonderful and I love you to bits. Thank you.

Notes

PROLOGUE

1 Jeremy Armstrong, "Change the Law for Max," *Mirror*, June 30, 2017.

2 Jeremy Armstrong, "At Last . . . Our Max Gets His New Heart," *Mirror*, September 1, 2017.

3 "2022 Organ Transplants Again Set National Records," United Network for Organ Sharing, January 10, 2023, https://unos.org/news/2022-organ-transplants-again-set-annual-records/.

4 "Organ Donation and Transplant Rates Continue to Recover, but Opportunities for Transplant Still Being Missed," NHS Blood and Transplant, July 12, 2023, https://www.nhsbt.nhs.uk/news/organ-donation-and-transplant-rates-continue-to-recover-but-opportunities-for-transplant-still-being-missed/.

5 Ibid.

6 James Randerson, "Woman Has Baby After First Ovary Transplant," *Guardian*, November 11, 2008.

7 Saami Khalifian et al., "Facial Transplantation: The First 9 Years," *Lancet* 384, no. 9960 (December 13, 2014): 2153–63.

8 Alok Jha, "Scientists Raise Hope for Sickle Cell Patients," *Guardian*, January 10, 2006.

9 "Transplant Cures Man of Diabetes," BBC, last updated March 9, 2005, http://news.bbc.co.uk/1/hi/health/4330717.stm.

10 "Family's Campaign to Create Organ Donor Register Has Helped Enable 18,000 Life-Saving and Life-Improving Transplants," NHS Blood and Transplant, June 18, 2018, https://www.nhsbt.nhs.uk/news/family-s-campaign-to-create-organ-donor-register-has-helped-enable-18-000-life-saving-and-life-improving-transplants/.

11 "NHS and Government Take Steps to Boost Organ Donation Registrations," NHS Blood and Transplant, September 22, 2023, https://www.organdonation.nhs.uk/get-involved/news/nhs-and-government-take-steps-to-boost-organ-donation-registrations/#:~:text=Meeting%20the%20need&text=As%20it%20stands%2030%20million,45%25%20of%20the%20total%20population.

12 Janet Radcliffe Richards, *The Ethics of Transplants* (Oxford, UK: Oxford University Press, 2012).

13 M. Mursal and Zahra Nader, "'I've Already Sold My Daughters; Now, My Kidney': Winter in Afghanistan's Slums," *Guardian*, January 23, 2022.

14 Matthew P. Robertson and Jacob Lavee, "Execution by Organ Procurement: Breaching the Dead Donor Rule in China," *American Journal of Transplantation* 22, no. 7 (July 2022): 1804–12.

15 Kazuo Ishiguro, *Never Let Me Go* (London: Faber and Faber, 2010).

16 Radcliffe Richards, *The Ethics of Transplants.*

KEIRA

1 "How Safe Are You on Britain's Main Road Networks?: British EuroRAP Results 2019," Road Safety Foundation, July 4, 2019, https://roadsafetyfoundation.org/how-safe-are-you-on-britains-main-road-networks/.

2 Neil Shaw, "Call for Government to Improve 'Dangerous' A361 Link Road After Three Serious Crashes," DevonLive, August 19, 2017, https://www.devonlive.com/news/devon-news/call-government-improve-dangerous-a361-296499.

3 "Children Killed with Mother in Devon Crash Were Twins," BBC, August 1, 2017, https://www.bbc.co.uk/news/uk-england-devon-40789659.

4 Natalie Gaskell et al., "Putting an End to Black Wednesday: Improving Patient Safety by Achieving Comprehensive Trust Induction and Mandatory Training by Day 1," *Clinical Medical* 16, no. 2 (April 2016): 124–28.

5 Randy Styner and Tony Farley, ed., *The Light of the Moon: Life, Death and the Birth of Advanced Trauma Life Support* (Raleigh, NC: Lulu Press, 2012).

6 Steven Bush, "A Trauma Course Born out of Personal Tragedy," Royal College of Surgeons of England, April 28, 2016, https://www.rcseng.ac.uk/news-and-events/blog/personal-tragedy/.

7 *ATLS Advanced Trauma Life Support: Student Course Manual*, 10th ed. (Chicago: American College of Surgeons, 2018).

8 Ibid.

9 J. K. Styner, "The Birth of Advanced Trauma Life Support (ATLS)," *Journal of Trauma Nursing* 13, no. 2 (2006): 41–44.

10 Ibid.

11 Ibid.

MAX

1 Desmond Sheridan, "The Heart, a Constant and Universal Metaphor," *European Heart Journal* 39, no. 37 (October 1, 2018): 3407–9.

2 Ambroise Paré, *The Workes of That Famous Chirurgion Ambrose Parey* (London: Th. Cotes and R. Young, 1634), available online at http://resource.nlm.nih.gov/2393053R.

3 Francesco Carelli, "The Book of Death: Weighing Your Heart," *London Journal of Primary Care* 4, no. 1 (July 2011): 86–87.

4 A. Rábano, "Aristotle's 'Mistake': The Structure and Function of the Brain in the Treatises on Biology," *Neurosciences and History* 6, no. 4 (2018): 138–43.

RESUSCITATION

1 Kyle J. Gunnerson et al., "Association of an Emergency Department-Based Intensive Care Unit with Survival and Inpatient Intensive Care Unit Admissions," *JAMA Network Open* 2, no. 7 (July 2019): e197584.

2   B. Ibsen, "The Anaesthetist's Viewpoint on the Treatment of Respiratory Complications in Poliomyelitis during the Epidemic in Copenhagen, 1952," *Proceedings of the Royal Society of Medicine* 47, no. 1 (January 1954): 72–74.

3   Robin S. Howard, "Poliomyelitis and the Postpolio Syndrome," *BMJ* 330, no. 7503 (June 4, 2005): 1314–18.

4   Philip Roth, *Nemesis* (London: Vintage, 2011).

5   David Oshinsky, *Polio: An American Story* (Oxford, UK: Oxford University Press, 2006).

6   Svetlana Bunimovich-Mendrazitsky and Lewi Stone, "Modeling Polio as a Disease of Development," *Journal of Theoretical Biology* 237, no. 3 (December 2005): 302–15.

7   "Infectious Diseases & Pandemics," *Harvard Public Health*, Fall 2013, https://www.hsph.harvard.edu/news/magazine/centennial-infectious-diseases-pandemics/.

8   Oshinsky, *Polio.*

9   H. Lassen, "A Preliminary Report on the 1952 Epidemic of Poliomyelitis in Copenhagen with Special Reference to the Treatment of Acute Respiratory Insufficiency," *Lancet* 1, no. 6749 (January 3, 1953): 37–41.

10 Ibid.

11 Louise Reisner-Sénélar, "The Birth of Intensive Care Medicine: Björn Ibsen's Records," *Intensive Care Medicine* 37, no. 7 (July 2011): 1084–86.

12 Caroline Richmond, "Bjørn Ibsen," *BMJ* 335, no. 7621 (September 2007): 674.

13 Bradley M. Wertheim, "How a Polio Outbreak in Copenhagen Led to the Invention of the Ventilator," *Smithsonian*, June 10, 2020, https://www.smithsonianmag.com/innovation/how-polio-outbreak-copenhagen-led-to-invention-ventilator-180975045/.

CROCODILES

1   "Ward 85–Tertiary Medical Ward," Manchester University NHS Foundation Trust, https://mft.nhs.uk/rmch/our-wards/ward-85-tertiary-medical-ward/.

2   "A Two Year Old Goes to Hospital (Robertson Films)," YouTube video, accessed June 30, 2023, https://www.youtube.com/watch?v=s14Q-_Bxc_U.

3   H. G. Monroe Davies, "Visits to Children in Hospital," *Spectator*, March 18, 1949, 362.

4   "A Two Year Old Goes to Hospital (Robertson Films)," YouTube.

5   L. Alsop-Shields and H. Mohay, "John Bowlby and James Robertson: Theorists, Scientists and Crusaders for Improvements in the Care of Children in Hospital," *Journal of Advanced Nursing* 35, no. 1 (July 2001): 50–58.

6   Ruth Davies, "Marking the 50th Anniversary of the Platt Report: From Exclusion, to Toleration and Parental Participation in the Care of the Hospitalized Child," *Journal of Child Health Care* 14, no. 1 (March 2010): 6–23.

7   E. M. R. Lomax, *Small and Special: The Development of Hospitals for Children in Victorian Britain* (London: Wellcome Institute for the History of Medicine, 1996).

8   Bruce Lindsay, "'A 2-Year-Old Goes to Hospital': A 50th Anniversary Reappraisal of the Impact of James Robertson's Film," *Journal of Child Health Care* 7, no. 1 (March 2003): 17–26.

9   Frank C. P. van der Horst and René van der Veer, "Changing Attitudes towards the Care of Children in Hospital: A New Assessment of the Influence of the Work of Bowlby and Robertson in the UK, 1940–1970," *Attachment & Human Development* 11, no. 2 (March 2009): 119–42.

10 John B. Watson, *Psychological Care of Infant and Child* (New York: Norton, 1928).
11 John Bowlby and James Robertson, "A Two-Year-Old Goes to Hospital," *Proceedings of the Royal Society of Medicine* 46, no. 6 (June 1953): 425–27.
12 van der Horst and van der Veer, "Changing Attitudes towards the Care of Children in Hospital."
13 Ibid.
14 James Robertson and Joyce Robertson, *Separation and the Very Young* (London: Free Association Books, 1989).
15 Ministry of Health, *The Welfare of Children in Hospital: Report by a Committee of the Central Health Services Council* (The Platt Report) (London: HMSO, 1959).
16 Sydney Brandon et al., "'What Is Wrong with Emotional Upset?'—50 Years on from the Platt Report," *Archives of Disease in Children* 94, no. 3 (March 2009): 173–77.
17 "Heart Heroes," Children's Heart Unit Fund, https://www.chuf.org.uk/about/heart-heroes/.
18 Institute of Transplantation, Newcastle: https://www.newcastle-hospitals.nhs.uk/hospitals/institute-of-transplantation/.
19 Claude S. Beck and Richmond L. Moore, "The Significance of the Pericardium in Relation to Surgery of the Heart," *Archives of Surgery* 11, no. 4 (1925): 550–77.
20 W. C. Aird, "Discovery of the Cardiovascular System: From Galen to William Harvey," *Journal of Thrombosis and Haemostasis* 9, suppl. 1 (July 2011): 118–29.
21 Debrah A. Wirtzfeld, "The History of Women in Surgery," *Canadian Journal of Surgery* 52, no. 4 (August 2009): 317–20.
22 Harold Ellis, "Suture of a Stab Wound of the Heart," *Journal of Perioperative Practice* 25, nos. 7–8 (July–August 2015): 144.
23 C. A. Elsberg, "An Experimental Investigation of the Treatment of Wounds of the Heart by Means of Suture of the Heart Muscle," *Journal of Experimental Medicine* 4, nos. 5–6 (September 1, 1899): 479–520.
24 Kjetil Söreide and Jon Arne Söreide, "Axel H. Cappelen, MD (1858–1919): First Suture of a Myocardial Laceration from a Cardiac Stab Wound," *Journal of Trauma and Acute Care Surgery* 60, no. 3 (March 2006): 653–54.
25 "Cardiac Surgery," *JAMA* 26, no. 24 (June 13, 1896): 1183–84.
26 Ibid.
27 Ibid.
28 Thomas Morris, *The Matter of the Heart: A History of the Heart in Eleven Operations* (London: Penguin, 2017).
29 Ibid.
30 "Surgery: The Ultimate Operation," *Time*, December 15, 1967.
31 Christiaan Barnard, *One Life* (Cape Town: Howard Timmins, 1969).

LIMBO

1 Graham Teasdale and Bryan Jennett, "Assessment of Coma and Impaired Consciousness. A Practical Scale," *Lancet* 2, no. 7872 (July 1974): 81–84.
2 Peter A. Meaney et al., "Cardiopulmonary Resuscitation Quality: Improving Cardiac Resuscitation Outcomes Both Inside and Outside the Hospital: A Consensus Statement from the American Heart Association," *Circulation* 128, no. 4 (July 23, 2013): 417–35.

3   R. S. Howard et al., "Hypoxic–Ischaemic Brain Injury: Imaging and Neurophysiology Abnormalities Related to Outcome," *QJM: An International Journal of Medicine* 105, no. 6 (June 2012): 551–61.

4   Marcin Sawicki et al., "CT Angiography in the Diagnosis of Brain Death," *Polish Journal of Radiology* 79 (November 15, 2014): 417–21.

5   "Thomas Willis: The Father of Neurology," Royal College of Physicians, https://history .rcplondon.ac.uk/blog/thomas-willis-father-neurology.

6   James P. B. O'Connor, "Thomas Willis and the Background to Cerebri Anatome," *Journal of the Royal Society of Medicine* 96, no. 3 (March 2003): 139–43.

7   Wilfred Owen, "Futility," Poetry Foundation, https://www.poetryfoundation.org /poems/57283/futility-56d23aa2d4b57.

8   Maurice A. Finocchiaro, *Defending Copernicus and Galileo: Critical Reasoning in the Two Affairs* (London: Springer, 2010).

9   Steven Laureys, "Death, Unconsciousness and the Brain," *Nature Reviews Neuroscience* 6, no. 11 (November 2005): 899–909.

10 B. K. Vitturi and W. L. Sanvito, "Pierre Mollaret (1898–1987)," *Journal of Neurology* 266 (2019): 1290–91.

11 P. Mollaret and M. Goulon, "Le Coma Dépassé," *Revue Neurologique* 101 (July 1959): 3–15.

12 William Spears, Asim Mian, and David Greer, "Brain Death: A Clinical Overview," *Journal of Intensive Care* 10, no. 1 (March 2022): 16.

13 Michael A. Kuiper and Erwin J. O. Kompanje, "Only a Very Bold Man Would Attempt to Define Death," *Intensive Care Medicine* 40 (March 2014): 897–99.

14 Radcliffe Richards, *The Ethics of Transplants*.

15 Linda A. Lewandowski, "Needs of Children during the Critical Illness of a Parent or Sibling," *Critical Care Nursing Clinics of North America* 4, no. 4 (December 1992): 573–85.

16 Janlyn R. Rozdilsky, "Enhancing Sibling Presence in Pediatric ICU," *Critical Care Nursing Clinics of North America* 17, no. 4 (December 2005): 451–61.

17 C. Kleiber, L. A. Montgomery, and M. Craft-Rosenberg, "Information Needs of the Siblings of Critically Ill Children," *Child Health Care* 24, no. 1 (Winter 1995): 47–60.

18 "Organ Donation for Transplantation: Improving Donor Identification and Consent Rates for Deceased Organ Donation," Clinical Guideline (CG135), NICE, published December 12, 2011, last updated December 21, 2016, https://www.nice .org.uk/guidance/cg135/chapter/1-Recommendations#identifying-patients-who -are-potential-donors.

HEARTWARE

1   "Nearly a Quarter of Children Waiting for an Organ Transplant Need a Heart," NHS Blood and Transplant press release, September 29, 2019, https://www.organdonation .nhs.uk/get-involved/news/nearly-a-quarter-of-children-waiting-for-an-organ -transplant-need-a-heart/.

2   A. Power et al., "Waitlist Mortality for Children Listed for Heart Transplant in the United States: How Are We Doing?," *Journal of Heart and Lung Transplantion* 40, no. 4 (April 2021): S37–S38.

3 "Heart Transplant FAQs," NHS Blood and Transplant, accessed February 24, 2023, https://www.nhsbt.nhs.uk/organ-transplantation/heart/is-a-heart-transplant-right -for-you/heart-transplant-faqs/.

4 "Annual Report on Cardiothoracic Organ Transplantation," NHS Blood and Transplant, September 2022, https://nhsbtdbe.blob.core.windows.net/umbraco-assets -corp/27816/nhsbt-annual-report-on-cardiothoracic-organ-transplantation-202122 .pdf.

5 L. C. Jordan et al., "Neurological Complications and Outcomes in the Berlin Heart EXCOR® Pediatric Investigational Device Exemption Trial," *Journal of the American Heart Association* 4, no. 1 (January 22, 2015): e001429.

6 Sung-Min Cho et al., "Cerebrovascular Events in Patients with Centrifugal-Flow Left Ventricular Assist Devices: Propensity Score-Matched Analysis from the Intermacs Registry," *Circulation* 144, no. 10 (September 7, 2021): 763–72.

7 Wirtzfeld, "The History of Women in Surgery."

8 Harold Ellis, "The Company of Barbers and Surgeons," *Journal of the Royal Society of Medicine* 94, no. 10 (October 2001): 548–49.

9 "The Week," *British Medical Journal* 2 (1862): 537.

10 Ourania Preventza and Leah Backhus, "US Women in Thoracic Surgery: Reflections on the Past and Opportunities for the Future," *Journal of Thoracic Disease* 13, no. 1 (January 29, 2021): 473–79.

11 Gervase Vernon, "Alexis Carrel: 'Father of Transplant Surgery' and Supporter of Eugenics," *British Journal of General Practice* 69, no. 684 (July 2019): 352.

12 P. Dutkowski, O. de Rougemont, and P.-A. Clavien, "Alexis Carrel: Genius, Innovator and Ideologist," *American Journal of Transplantation* 8, no. 10 (October 2008): 1998–2003.

13 Paul Craddock, *Spare Parts: A Surprising History of Transplants* (New York: St. Martin's Press, 2022).

14 A. W. H. Bates, "Vivisection, Virtue, and the Law in the Nineteenth Century," 13–42, in *Anti-Vivisection and the Profession of Medicine in Britain* (London: Palgrave Macmillan, 2017).

15 Robert M. Sade, "Transplantation at 100 Years: Alexis Carrel, Pioneer Surgeon," *Annals of Thoracic Surgery* 80, no. 6 (December 2005): 2415–18.

16 Craddock, *Spare Parts*.

17 Alexis Carrel, "La technique opératoire des anastomoses vasculaire et la transplantation des viscères," *Lyon Medical* 99 (1902): 859–62.

18 David Hamilton, *A History of Organ Transplantation: Ancient Legends to Modern Practice* (Pittsburgh: University of Pittsburgh Press, 2012).

19 E. A. Bonfils-Roberts, "The Rib Spreader: A Chapter in the History of Thoracic Surgery," *Chest* 61, no. 5 (May 1972): 469–74.

20 C. E. Baisden, L. V. Greenwald, and P. N. Symbas, "Occult Rib Fractures and Brachial Plexus Injury following Median Sternotomy for Open-Heart Operations," *Annals of Thoracic Surgery* 38, no. 3 (September 1984): 192–94.

21 Thet Su Win and James Henderson, "Management of Traumatic Amputations of the Upper Limb," *BMJ* 348, clinical review ed. (February 15, 2014): 29–32.

22 Myriam Lacerte, Angela Hays Shapshak, and Fassil B. Mesfin, *Hypoxic Brain Injury* (Treasure Island, FL: StatPearls, 2023), available from https://www.ncbi.nlm.nih.gov /books/NBK537310/.

23 A. J. Gunn et al., "Therapeutic Hypothermia Translates from Ancient History into Practice," *Pediatric Research* 81, nos. 1–2 (January 2017): 202–9.

24 Wilfred G. Bigelow, *Cold Hearts: The Story of Hypothermia and the Pacemaker in Heart Surgery* (Toronto: McClelland and Stewart, 1984).

25 Ivan Oransky, "Wilfred Gordon Bigelow," *Lancet* 365, no. 9471 (May 2005): 1616.

26 Lawrence H. Cohn, "Fifty Years of Open-Heart Surgery," *Circulation* 107, no. 17 (May 6, 2003): 2168–70.

27 J. H. Gibbon Jr., "The Gestation and Birth of an Idea," *Philadelphia Medicine* 59 (1963): 913–16.

28 Tom P. Theruvath and John S. Ikonomidis, "Historical Perspectives of the American Association for Thoracic Surgery: John H. Gibbon, Jr. (1903–1973)," *Journal of Thoracic and Cardiovascular Surgery* 147, no. 3 (March 2014): 833–36.

29 Cohn, "Fifty Years of Open-Heart Surgery."

30 Matthias Ochs et al., "The Number of Alveoli in the Human Lung," *American Journal of Respiratory and Critical Care Medicine* 169, no. 1 (January 1, 2004): 120–24.

31 Eleonore Fröhlich et al., "Measurements of Deposition, Lung Surface Area and Lung Fluid for Simulation of Inhaled Compounds," *Frontiers in Pharmacology* 7 (June 24, 2016): 181.

32 Morris, *The Matter of the Heart.*

33 Jordan, P. Bloom et al., "John H. Gibbon, Jr., M.D.: Surgical Innovator, Pioneer, and Inspiration," *American Surgery* 77, no. 9 (September 2011): 1112–14.

34 Hans Meisner, "Milestones in Surgery: 60 Years of Open Heart Surgery," *Journal of Thoracic and Cardiovascular Surgery* 62, no. 8 (December 2014): 645–50.

35 N. Shumway, "Clarence Walton Lillehei," *BMJ* 319, no. 7213 (September 25, 1999): 856.

36 V. L. Gott and N. E. Shumway, "Cross-Circulation: A Milestone in Cardiac Surgery," *Journal of Thoracic and Cardiovascular Surgery* 127, no. 3 (March 2004): 617.

37 H. E. Warden, "C. Walton Lillehei: Pioneer Cardiac Surgeon," *Journal of Thoracic and Cardiovascular Surgery* 98, no. 5, pt. 2 (November 1989): 833–45.

38 Ibid.

39 Denton A. Cooley, "The Key That Opened the Door: 50 Years of Open Heart Surgery," *Texas Heart Institute Journal* 31, no. 3 (2004): 206.

40 Barnard, *One Life.*

MATCHING

1 E. J. Cameron et al., "Confirmation of Brainstem Death," *Practical Neurology* 16, no. 2 (April 2016): 129–35.

2 "Donation after Death Using Neurological Criteria—Donor Optimisation Care Bundle," NHS Blood and Transplant, June 13, 2023, https://nhsbtdbe.blob.core .windows.net/umbraco-assets-corp/29992/frm7261.docx.

3 Peter Medawar, *Memoir of a Thinking Radish* (Oxford, UK: Oxford University Press,1986).

4 T. E. Starzl, "Peter Brian Medawar: Father of Transplantation," *Journal of the American College of Surgeons* 180, no. 3 (March 1995): 332–36.

5   Medawar, *Memoir of a Thinking Radish.*

6   Ibid.

7   Ibid.

8   T. Gibson and P. B. Medawar, "The Fate of Skin Homografts in Man," *Journal of Anatomy* 77, pt. 4 (July 1943): 299–310.

9   Dutkowski et al., "Alexis Carrel."

10 W. J. Dempster, B. Lennox, J. W. Boag, "Prolongation of Survival of Skin Homotransplants in the Rabbit by Irradiation of the Host," *British Journal of Experimental Pathology* 31 (1950): 670–79; John A. Morgan, "The Influence of Cortisone on the Survival of Homografts of Skin in the Rabbit," *Surgery* 30, no. 3 (September 1951): 506–15.

11 Starzl, "Peter Brian Medawar."

12 R. E. Billingham, L. Brent, and P. B. Medawar, "'Actively Acquired Tolerance' of Foreign Cells," *Nature* 172, no. 4379 (October 3, 1953): 603–6.

13 Starzl, "Peter Brian Medawar."

14 Ibid.

15 "Organ Donation and Transplantation," NHS Blood and Transplant, accessed September 2, 2023, https://www.nhsbt.nhs.uk/what-we-do/transplantation-services /organ-donation-and-transplantation/#:~:text=Thanks%20to%20our%20amazing%20 donors,while%20waiting%20for%20a%20transplant.

16 "Organ Donation Statistics," Health Resources & Services Administration, accessed September 2, 2023, https://www.organdonor.gov/learn/organ-donation-statistics.

17 María Jesús Valero-Masa et al., "Cold Ischemia >4 Hours Increases Heart Transplantation Mortality: An Analysis of the Spanish Heart Transplantation Registry," *International Journal of Cardiology* 319 (November 15, 2020): 14–19.

WAITING

1   Domingo Liotta et al., "Prolonged Assisted Circulation during and after Cardiac or Aortic Surgery. Prolonged Partial Left Ventricular Bypass by Means of Intracorporeal Circulation," *American Journal of Cardiology* 12 (September 1963): 399–405; Domingo Liotta, "Early Clinical Application of Assisted Circulation," *Texas Heart Institute Journal* 29, no. 3 (February 2002): 229–30.

2   David K. C. Cooper, *Open Heart: The Radical Surgeons Who Revolutionized Medicine* (New York: Kaplan, 2010).

3   M. E. DeBakey and W. C. Roberts, "Michael Ellis DeBakey: A Conversation with the Editor. Interview by William C. Roberts," *American Journal of Cardiology* 79, no. 7 (April 1, 1997): 929–50.

4   Cooper, *Open Heart.*

5   M. E. DeBakey, "Left Ventricular Bypass Pump for Cardiac Assistance: Clinical Experience," *American Journal of Cardiology* 27, no. 1 (January 1971): 3–11.

6   "Surgery's New Frontier," *Time*, March 25, 1957.

7   "The Best Hope of All," *Time*, May 3, 1963.

8   Caroline Richmond, "Norman Shumway: The Father of Heart Transplantation and Surgeon Who Performed the World's First Heart-Lung Transplant," *BMJ* 332, no. 7540 (March 4, 2006): 553.

9   Donald McRae, *Every Second Counts: The Extraordinary Race to Transplant the First Human Heart* (London: Simon & Schuster, 2006).

10 N. E. Shumway and R. R. Lower, "Topical Cardiac Hypothermia for Extended Periods of Anoxic Arrest," *Surgical Forum* 10 (1960): 563–66.

11 N. E. Shumway, R. R. Lower, and R. C. Stofer, "Selective Hypothermia of the Heart in Anoxic Cardiac Arrest," *Surgery, Gynecology & Obstetrics* 109 (December 1959): 750–54.

12 R. R. Lower and N. E. Shumway, "Studies on Orthotopic Homotransplantation of The Canine Heart," *Surgical Forum* 11 (1960): 18–19.

13 Charles P. Bieber, Edward B. Stinson, and Norman E. Shumway, "Pathology of the Conduction System in Cardiac Rejection," *Circulation* 39, no. 5 (May 1969): 567–75.

14 J. S. Shroeder et al., "Acute Rejection following Cardiac Transplantation: Phonocardiographic and Ultrasound Observations," *Circulation* 40, no. 2 (August 1969): 155–64.

15 Richmond, "Norman Shumway."

16 Ivan Oransky, "Norman Shumway," *Lancet* 367, no. 9514 (March 18, 2006): 875.

17 Jeremy Armstrong, "Change the Law for Max," *Mirror*, June 30, 2017.

GOODBYE

1   "The National Organ Retrieval Service and Usage of Organs," NHS Blood and Transport, accessed September 9, 2023, https://nhsbtdbe.blob.core.windows.net /umbraco-assets-corp/24042/section-4-the-national-organ-retrieval-service-and -usage-of-organs.pdf.

JUDGMENT

1   J. Pegrum and O. Pearce, "A Stressful Job: Are Surgeons Psychopaths?," *Bulletin of the Royal College of Surgeons of England* 97, no. 8 (September 2015): 331–34.

2   Ibid.

3   F. Tonnaer et al., "Screening for Psychopathy: Validation of the Psychopathic Personality Inventory–Short Form with Reference Scores," *Journal of Psychopathology and Behavioral Assessment* 35, no. 2 (2013): 153–61.

4   Stephen Westaby and Henry Marsh, "What Makes a Great Surgeon? Two of Britain's Best Discuss," *Financial Times*, September 8, 2017.

5   Stephen Westaby, *Fragile Lives: A Heart Surgeon's Stories of Life and Death on the Operating Table* (London: HarperCollins, 2017).

6   Cooper, *Open Heart*.

7   Tonnaer et al., "Screening for Psychopathy."

8   Joshua D. Mezrich, *How Death Becomes Life: Notes from a Transplant Surgeon* (London: Atlantic Books, 2019).

9   Louis H. Toledo-Pereyra, "Christiaan Barnard," *Journal of Investigative Surgery* 23, no. 2 (May 2010): 72–78.

10 McRae, *Every Second Counts*.

11 Raymond Hoffenberg, "Christiaan Barnard: His First Transplants and Their Impact on Concepts of Death," *BMJ* 323, no. 7327 (December 22, 2001): 1478–80.

12 Barnard, *One Life*; B. Cupido and M. Ntsekhe, "The Groote Schuur Cardiac Clinic: A Centre of Cardiovascular Excellence at the Tip of the African Continent," *European Heart Journal* 40, no. 5 (2019): 406–8.

13 Barnard, *One Life*.

14 Mollaret and Goulon, "Le Coma Dépassé"; Spears et al., "Brain Death: A Clinical Overview."

15 McRae, *Every Second Counts*.

16 David K. C. Cooper, "Christiaan Barnard—The Surgeon Who Dared: The Story of the First Human-to-Human Heart Transplant," *Global Cardiology Science and Practice* 2018, no. 2 (June 30, 2018): 11.

17 James-Brent Styan, *Heartbreaker: Christiaan Barnard and the First Heart Transplant* (Cape Town: Jonathan Ball, 2017).

18 Barnard, *One Life*.

19 McRae, *Every Second Counts*.

20 Jillian Hurst, "A Modern Cosmas and Damian: Sir Roy Calne and Thomas Starzl Receive the 2012 Lasker-DeBakey Clinical Medical Research Award," *Journal of Clinical Investigation* 122, no. 10 (September 2012): 3378–82.

21 Roy Calne, "Heart Transplants in the Headlines," *Lancet* 373, no. 9671 (April 2009): 1241–42.

22 "Surgery: The Ultimate Operation," *Time*, December 15, 1967, https://content.time .com/time/subscriber/article/0,33009,837606,00.html.

23 "The Heart Savers," *Sunday Times Weekly Review*, December 10, 1967.

24 Barnard, *One Life*.

25 Ibid.

26 Cicely Saunders, "The Evolution of Palliative Care," *Journal of the Royal Society of Medicine* 94, no. 9 (September 2001): 430–32.

27 D. J. Rowe, "Dr. Christiaan Barnard: Renowned Surgeon, Egoist but an Old-Fashioned Family Doctor at Heart. Interview by Robert MacNeil," *Canadian Medical Association Journal* 120, no. 1 (January 6, 1979): 98–99.

28 Ayesha Nathoo, *Hearts Exposed: Transplants and the Media in 1960s Britain* (Basingstoke, UK: Palgrave Macmillian, 2009).

29 Calne, "Heart Transplants in the Headlines."

30 J. D. Haller and M. M. Cerruti, "Heart Transplantation in Man: Compilation of Cases, January 1, 1964 to October 23, 1968," *American Journal of Cardiology* 22, no. 6 (December 1968): 840–43.

31 Nathoo, *Hearts Exposed*.

32 "Heart Operation Held in Secrecy," *Guardian*, May 4, 1968.

33 D. A. Cooley, "In Memoriam: Donald N. Ross (1922–2014)," *Texas Heart Institute Journal* 41, no. 5 (2014): 456–57.

34 Malcolm Gladwell and David Epstein, "10,000 Hours vs. The Sports Gene," MIT Sloan Sports Analytics Conference 2014 video, accessed September 12, 2023, https:// www.youtube.com/watch?v=iXBhINPoKEk&t=787s.

35 Malcolm Gladwell, *Outliers: The Story of Success* (London: Little, Brown, 2008).

36 John Haggie (@Johnrockdoc), "5y learning how, 5y learning when, n a lifetime learning when not to operate," Twitter, March 1, 2014, https://twitter.com/Johnrockdoc/status /439839702409961472.

37 Barry Jackson, "What Makes an Excellent Surgeon?," *Obesity Surgery* 29 (March 2019): 1087–89.

38 Alan J. Hawk, "ArtiFacts: Built for Speed—Robert Liston's Surgical Technique," Clinical Orthopaedics and Related Research 479, no. 4 (April 2021): 679–80.
39 Jackson, "What Makes an Excellent Surgeon?"

RETRIEVAL

1 Barnard, *One Life*.
2 "Organ Donation as Part of End-of-Life Care," ODT Clinical, accessed September 12, 2023, https://www.odt.nhs.uk/deceased-donation/best-practice-guidance/end-of-life-care/.
3 Raymond Pfister et al., "Heart Procurement in a Multi-Organ Donor," Multimedia Manual of Cardio-Thoracic Surgery, accessed September 12, 2023, https://mmcts.org/tutorial/1438.
4 Alia Dani et al., "Effect of Ischemic Time on Pediatric Heart Transplantation Outcomes: Is It the Same for All Allografts?," *Pediatric Transplantation* 26, no. 4 (June 2022): e14259.
5 Andrew K. Burroughs et al., "3-Month and 12-Month Mortality after First Liver Transplant in Adults in Europe: Predictive Models for Outcome," *Lancet* 367, no. 9506 (January 21, 2006): 225–32.
6 Germaine Wong et al., "The Impact of Total Ischemic Time, Donor Age and the Pathway of Donor Death on Graft Outcomes after Deceased Donor Kidney Transplantation," *Transplantation* 101, no. 6 (June 2017): 1152–58.
7 Caroline Kettlewell, "When Minutes Matter," United Network for Organ Sharing, February 15, 2023, https://unos.org/news/insights/when-minutes-matter-organ-transportation/.
8 JoNel Aleccia, "Lost Luggage: How Lifesaving Organs for Transplant Go Missing in Transit," NBC News, February 8, 2020, https://www.nbcnews.com/health/health-news/lost-luggage-how-lifesaving-organs-transplant-go-missing-transit-n1130891.
9 Kirk Johnson, "A Human Heart, Left Aboard, Sends Airplane Back to Where It Started," *New York Times*, December 13, 2018.
10 Aleccia, "Lost Luggage."

TRANSPLANT

1 *Heart Transplant: A Chance to Live*, BBC Two, broadcast May 19, 2018.
2 Ibid.
3 Simon Blackburn, *Oxford Dictionary of Philosophy* (Oxford, UK: Oxford University Press, 2008).
4 Barnard, *One Life*.
5 *Heart Transplant: A Chance to Live*, BBC Two.

AFTERMATH

1 Shunsuke Saito et al., "Successful Treatment of Cardiogenic Shock Caused by Humoral Cardiac Allograft Rejection," *Circulation Journal* 73, no. 5 (May 2009): 970–73.
2 Henry T. Tribe, "The Discovery and Development of Cyclosporin," *Mycologist* 12, no. 1 (February 1998): 20–22.
3 Jamil R. Azzi, Mohamed H. Sayegh, and Samir G. Mallat, "Calcineurin Inhibitors: 40 Years Later, Can't Live Without . . . ," *Journal of Immunology* 191, no. 12 (December 15, 2013): 5785–91.

4 Roy Calne, "Cyclosporine as a Milestone in Immunosuppression," *Transplantation Proceedings* 36, suppl. 2 (March 2004): 13S–15S.

5 Gina Kolata, "Drug Transforms Transplant Medicine," *Science* 221, no. 4605 (July 1, 1983): 40–42.

6 Jamie Talan, "Scientist's Holiday Leads to New Drug," *New York Times*, February 12, 1984.

7 Jeremy Armstrong, "'Our Sister's Heart Lives On in Max': Emotional Meeting between Family of Tragic Girl and the Transplant Boy Whose Life She Saved," *Mirror*, May 1, 2018.

EPILOGUE

1 "Max and Keira's Law Comes into Effect in England," NHS Blood and Transplant, May 20, 2020, https://www.organdonation.nhs.uk/get-involved/news/max-and-keira -s-law-comes-into-effect-in-england/.

2 "Organ Donation (Deemed Consent) Act 2019, Volume 696: Debated on Tuesday 8 June 2021," Hansard, UK Parliament, https://hansard.parliament.uk/commons /2021-06-08/debates/8E86ABBA-EBD2-4348-AB33-490BEBCE72DF /OrganDonation(DeemedConsent)Act2019#:~:text=The%20organ%20donation%20 opt%2Dout,that%20took%20place%20last%20year.

3 "Organ and Tissue Donation and Transplantation Activity Report 2022/23," NHS Blood and Transplant, https://nhsbtdbe.blob.core.windows.net/umbraco-assets-corp /30198/activity-report-2022-2023-final.pdf.

4 Wojciech Zakrzewski et al., "Stem Cells: Past, Present, and Future," *Stem Cell Research & Therapy* 10, no. 1 (February 26, 2019): 68.